Adult Congenital Heart Disease

A PRACTICAL GUIDE

D0932693

To our parents for bringing us to life,
our teachers for helping us see,
our spouses for their understanding and
our children, the very best thing that we have.

DREXEL UNIVERSITY
HEALTH SCIENCES LIBRARIES
HAHNEMANN LIBRARY

Adult Congenital Heart Disease

A PRACTICAL GUIDE

Michael A. Gatzoulis
Royal Brompton Hospital *and*
National Heart & Lung Institute at the Imperial College
London, UK

Lorna Swan
Department of Cardiology
Western Infirmary
Glasgow, UK

Judith Therrien
Sir M. Davis Jewish General Hospital
McGill University
Montreal, Quebec, Canada

George A. Pantely
Division of Cardiology
Oregon Health and Science University
Portland, Oregon, USA

INCLUDING
'Pregnancy and Contraception' chapter
by Philip J. Steer

FOREWORD BY
Eugene Braunwald

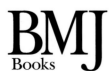

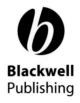

Blackwell
Publishing

WG
220
A2445
2005

© 2005 by Blackwell Publishing Ltd
BMJ Books is an imprint of the BMJ Publishing Group Limited, used under licence

Blackwell Publishing, Inc., 350 Main Street, Malden, Massachusetts 02148-5020, USA
Blackwell Publishing Ltd, 9600 Garsington Road, Oxford OX4 2DQ, UK
Blackwell Publishing Asia Pty Ltd, 550 Swanston Street, Carlton, Victoria 3053, Australia

The right of the Authors to be identified as the Authors of this Work has been asserted in accordance
with the Copyright, Designs and Patents Act 1988.

All rights reserved. No part of this publication may be reproduced, stored in a retrieval system,
or transmitted, in any form or by any means, electronic, mechanical, photocopying, recording or
otherwise, except as permitted by the UK Copyright, Designs and Patents Act 1988, without the prior
permission of the publisher.

First published 2005

Library of Congress Cataloging-in-Publication Data

Adult congenital heart disease : a practical guide / Michael A. Gatzoulis ... [et al.] ; foreword by Eugene
Braunwald
     p. ; cm.
   Includes index.
   ISBN 0-7279-1668-8
1. Congenital heart disease.
   [DNLM: 1. Heart Defects, Congenital—Adult. WG 220 A2445 2005] I. Gatzoulis, Michael A.

   RC687.A454 2005
   616.1'2043—dc22

                                                                                2004019723

ISBN 0-7279-1668-8

A catalogue record for this title is available from the British Library

Commissioning Editor: Mary Banks
Development Editor: Nick Morgan
Project Manager: Tom Fryer, Sparks
Production Controller: Kate Charman

Set in Palatino 9.5/12pt by Sparks, Oxford – www.sparks.co.uk
Printed and bound in India by Replika Press Pvt. Ltd

For further information on Blackwell Publishing, visit our website:
http://www.blackwellpublishing.com

The publisher's policy is to use permanent paper from mills that operate a sustainable forestry policy,
and which has been manufactured from pulp processed using acid-free and elementary chlorine-
free practices. Furthermore, the publisher ensures that the text paper and cover board used have met
acceptable environmental accreditation standards.

Contents

Foreword

The diagnosis and successful management of congenital heart disease represents one of the greatest triumphs of cardiovascular medicine and surgery in the 20th century. As a consequence, the number of adults with congenital heart disease – both with repaired and unrepaired lesions – has grown rapidly, and is now approaching one million in North America. Similar increases have occurred in Western Europe. The care of adults with congenital heart disease represents a major challenge. They include a large number of diverse anatomic malformations of varying severities at various stages of their natural history and with different degrees of anatomic repair. Approximately one-third of these patients are considered to have 'simple' congenital heart disease, such as mild pulmonic stenosis or repaired ventricular septal defect. The majority, however, such as those with cyanotic congenital heart disease, have lesions of greater complexity.

The growing population of adults with congenital heart disease presents unique problems in management. Arrhythmias are frequent and are often of serious import. Pregnancy presents special problems. The risk of infective endocarditis and premature ventricular dysfunction may occur in patients even following successful correction. There is a delicate interplay between managing the usual risks for the development of coronary artery disease in adults and the residua of repaired congenital heart disease, such as coarctation of the aorta.

During the past two decades the approach to the diagnosis and treatment of adults with congenital heart disease has been totally transformed. For many years the catheterization laboratory was the site of diagnosis while the operating room the site of treatment. Now, the imaging laboratory is the primary diagnostic site and increasingly invasive treatment is carried out in the catheterization laboratory.

Ideally, adults with congenital heart disease should be cared for at regional adult congenital heart disease centers, staffed by cardiologists trained in both pediatric and adult cardiology, who are trained in the special problems presented by these patients. Regional centers alone, however, cannot do the whole job. Cardiologists not specifically trained to care for patients with congenital heart disease, other physicians and allied health professionals outside these regional centers are required to participate in the care of these patients. *Adult Congenital Heart Disease: A Practical Guide* by Gatzoulis, Swan, Therrien and Pantely will be a valued resource to these practitioners. This guide describes the various forms of congenital heart disease in sufficient detail to allow the practitioner to diagnose and manage most of their problems, yet it is not the encyclopedic text required by the subspecialist and often overwhelming to the non-specialist. The sections on general principles, including pregnancy, contraception, infective endocarditis, anticoagulation, arrhythmias, syncope, heart failure and the care of the cyanosed patient, are particularly well written.

There has been fear that the adult with congenital heart disease could fall between the cracks and become a medical orphan. *Adult Congenital Heart Disease: A Practical Guide* will become an important educational resource to help diminish this fear.

Eugene Braunwald, MD
Boston, MA, USA

Preface

Congenital heart disease with an approximate incidence of 1% is the most common inborn defect, which used to carry a very poor prognosis. Advances in diagnosis and management of patients with congenital heart disease over the latter part of the 20th century, however, have led to the majority of such patients surviving to adulthood. There are currently hundreds of thousands of individuals around the world who either have survived life-saving childhood surgery or are diagnosed with congenital heart disease in later life—often during pregnancy. Most of these patients have ongoing lifelong congenital heart and other medical needs. They are regularly seen by their family physicians and, increasingly, by office and hospital specialists, presenting both a significant workload and a management challenge. While patients with congenital heart disease represent, therefore, a common challenge to health care, there has been and continues to be a marked shortfall in training programs and in resource allocation to provide for them.

It is the aim of this smaller textbook to introduce this important subject to a larger audience, namely general physicians, non-congenital heart specialists, health allied professionals and trainees, all of whom are now involved with the care of the congenital heart patient. Our main focus has been to introduce general principles in recognizing the problem, discuss management of common lesions and provide essential information on dealing with emergencies. Our ultimate goal was to familiarize the various disciplines involved with this important subject and facilitate appropriate and timely specialist referral of the congenital heart patient. Knowledge is power, and it is hoped that better informed health professionals (and patients) will improve further the longer-term prospects of what is considered to be one of the most successful endeavors of modern medicine.

Michael A. Gatzoulis
Lorna Swan
Judith Therrien
George A. Pantely

Acknowledgments

The authors are deeply indebted to their colleagues Professor Philip Steer for the pregnancy and contraception chapter, Professor Leon Gerlis for his morphologic drawings, Drs Philip Kilner, Wei Li and Yen Ho for their cardiac MRI, echocardiographic and morphologic specimens, Drs Jack Colman, Erwin Oechslin and Dylan Taylor for allowing us to use the congenital heart glossary, Dr Craig Broberg for the appendix on shunt calculations, and to Mary Banks, Nick Morgan, Tom Fryer and the BMJ Books/Blackwell team for their enthusiastic support throughout the project. Dr Gatzoulis and the Royal Brompton Adult Congenital Heart Program are supported by the British Heart Foundation.

PART 1

General Principles

CHAPTER 1

Epidemiology of Congenital Heart Disease

A 'congenital' heart disease is by definition a disease that has been present since birth. However, many congenital clinics may see a wider variety of defects that were either not present or not evident from birth.

Those present but not usually detected in early life include lesions such as a moderate size atrial septal defect. Others, that are only anatomically present in later years with a latent predisposition prior to this, such as many of the cardiomyopathies, are not strictly 'congenital' but are often included in this patient group.

Approximately 60% of all congenital heart disease is diagnosed in babies less than a year old, 30% in children and 10% in adults (those over 16 years of age). However, there are now more adults than children with congenital lesions and this has important implications for those practicing in any branch of adult medicine.

The majority of adults with congenital heart lesions will make their way to the adult practitioner via the pediatric cardiologist. These patients have been the beneficiaries of advances in pediatric cardiology and cardiac surgery services, exemplified by the fact that 96% of children with congenital cardiac lesions who survive infancy will live to at least 15 years of age.

The live birth incidence of congenital heart disease is approximately 7 confirmed cases per 1000 or 1 in every 145 babies born. This figure obviously varies according to the population studied but is an approximation for many Western countries. This value has been affected little by antenatal diagnosis. The prevalence of congenital heart lesions is more difficult to determine, especially in adults. In the UK (with a population of approximately 60 million) it is thought there are at least 150,000 adults with congenital heart disease. This would be equivalent to a prevalence of 250 cases per 100,000. (See Table 1.1.)

Ventricular septal defect	30%	**Table 1.1** Commonest cardiac lesions (at birth)
Atrial septal defect	10%	
Patent ductus	10%	
Pulmonary stenosis	7%	
Coarctation	7%	
Aortic stenosis	6%	
Tetralogy of Fallot	6%	
D-transposition	4%	
Other	20%	

Nomenclature

One of the main 'turn-offs' for the non-specialist regarding congenital heart disease is the confusing and apparently cumbersome nomenclature used. A prime example of this is the multiple terms used for a single condition, e.g. double discordance, L-transposition of the great arteries, or congenitally corrected transposition.

Unfortunately, detailed descriptive nomenclature is vital to the understanding of the anatomy, physiology and outcome of these patients. Segmental logical description should hopefully minimize confusion but it is still difficult for the non-specialist to unravel the implications of these terms. In many of these cases a picture speaks a thousand words, and in combination with a helpful congenital cardiologist at the end of the phone most of the pertinent details can be effectively communicated. A glossary and a list of helpful websites that also help explain cardiac anatomy are included towards the end of this book.

Etiology

The crucial period for fetal cardiac development occurs between weeks 6 and 12. In addition, ductal abnormalities, valve lesions and abnormalities of the myocardium can occur later in pregnancy. Clinically, patients want to know:
1 Why did this happen? and
2 Will it happen again (i.e. will other siblings and future offspring be affected)?

The etiology of congenital lesions can be separated into genetic and non-genetic. Non-genetic causes (Table 1.2) would include illness in the mother (such as rubella or diabetes) or maternal drug ingestion (including anti-epileptics, alcohol, and lithium). Examples of common deletions and duplications are shown in Table 1.3.

Approximately 17% of congenital cardiac conditions occur in association with a recognized syndrome that 'causes' the defect. However, the genetic contribution to congenital heart lesions is much greater. Over the last decade numerous genetic loci and chromosomal abnormalities have been identified for a whole range of conditions. One only needs to look at the recurrence rate

Table 1.2 Non-genetic etiology of congenital lesions and cardiac involvement

Non-genetic etiology	Cardiac involvement
Maternal rubella	Patent ductus arteriosus, pulmonary stenosis, arterial stenoses, atrial septal defect
Lithium	Tricuspid valve disease
Fetal alcohol syndrome	Ventricular septal defect
Maternal lupus	Congenital heart block

Table 1.3 Examples of common deletions/duplications

Hypoplastic left heart syndrome	11q23–25 deletion
Coarctation	4q31, 5q23–31 deletions
Tetralogy of Fallot	22q11, 8p22 deletions

for mothers with congenital heart disease to realize that familial and genetic factors contribute to many of the most common lesions (see Chapter 3 for recurrence rates).

Pediatric books list a plethora of rare congenital cardiac syndromes. Many of these are associated with multisystem involvement. The more complex of these lesions often result in the deaths of these children before they reach the adult practitioner. Table 1.4 lists some of the more common lesions the adult physician or surgeon might see.

Table 1.4 Some of the more common lesions seen by the adult physician

Syndrome	Cardiac manifestation	Non-cardiac manifestations
Holt-Oram	Septation defects (ASD, VSD)	Limb reduction defects Autosomal dominant – 12q35 TBXS transcription factor
Ellis-Van Creveld	Single atrium ASD	Limb and nail defects
Noonan	Pulmonary valve dysplasia Cardiomyopathy (hypertrophic, often right-sided)	Web neck, short stature, pectus, cryptorchism
Turner	Coarctation Bicuspid aortic valve	Chromosome XO Lymphedema Short stature Web neck
Kartagener	Dextrocardia	Situs inversus, sinusitis, bronchiectasis
LEOPARD	Pulmonary stenosis	Multiple lentigines Deaf, nevi, rib abnormalities

Commoner congenital cardiac syndromes

Several syndromes deserve specific mention, either due to their frequency or because of important non-cardiac features.

Trisomy 21 (Down syndrome)

The association between trisomy 21 and congenital heart disease is well recognized. Babies with Down syndrome and an atrioventricular septal defect (AVSD) should undergo early repair prior to the development of pulmonary hypertension. However, in the past, different long-term survival rates for Down syndrome per se and higher perioperative mortality were thought to be barriers to cardiac repair, resulting in a number of adult patients with trisomy 21 and an AVSD who have undergone reparative surgery. In the adult population it is not, therefore, uncommon to see patients with Down syndrome with cyanosis and secondary erthyrocytosis.

Atrioventricular septal defects (often complete defects with an atrial and ventricular septal defect and AV valve abnormalities, see Chapter 10) and tetralogy of Fallot are the most common cardiac lesions. Down syndrome coexists in 35% of patients with an AVSD and in >75% of those with complete AVSD.

In caring for these adults, other important components of their Down syndrome that may impact on their cardiac status include their tendency to obstructive sleep apnea and thyroid disease.

DiGeorge syndrome (CATCH 22)

DiGeorge syndrome or CATCH 22 is due to deletion of chromosome 22 (22q11 deletion). This is a relatively common genetic defect amongst congenital heart patients. Approximately 15% of patients with tetralogy have this deletion. This is more likely if they also have a right-sided aortic arch, pulmonary atresia or aortic-to-pulmonary collaterals. Other components of the 22q11 deletion syndrome include (Cardiac defect) Abnormal facies, Thymic hypoplasia, Cleft palate and Hypocalcemia (hence the name CATCH 22). This genetic defect usually occurs sporadically, but affected subjects have a 50% risk of passing the defect to their offspring. There is a simple (although not 100% diagnostic) FISH blood test for DiGeorge syndrome and this should be offered to all patients with tetralogy who are considering pregnancy.

Other cardiac conditions commonly found in 22q11 deletion include interrupted aortic arch and truncus arteriosus. 22q11 patients also have a higher risk of psychiatric disorder, usually depression, that can influence their quality of life and compliance with cardiac follow-up.

Williams syndrome

Williams syndrome is associated with cardiac, neurodevelopmental and multisystem abnormalities and is caused by a deletion of chromosome 7q11.23. The most common cardiac abnormalities are supravalvar aortic stenosis, peripheral pulmonary artery stenoses and other arterial abnormalities such as coronary artery ostial stenoses. Left-sided lesions tend to progress (supraval-var aortic stenosis), whereas right-sided abnormalities (pulmonary) are often static or may progress spontaneously. Subjects with Williams syndrome have also abnormalities of calcium metabolism, hence hypocalcemia—usually neo-natal—may be a clinical problem.

Long-term outcome

Lesion-specific long-term outcome data will be discussed in following chapters.

Mortality from congenital heart disease has declined dramatically in babies and children. The vast majority of these children are now expected to reach adult life. In the UK, in 1986 60% of deaths from congenital heart disease occurred in babies less than a year old. By the 1990s this picture had dramatically changed and now the majority of congenital heart deaths occur in adults over the age of 20.

Further reading

Hoffman JIE & Kaplan S (2002) The incidence of congenital heart disease. *Journal of the American College of Cardiology,* **39**, 1890–1900.

Petersen S, Peto V & Rayner M (2003) *Congenital heart disease statistics 2003*. British Heart Foundation Health Promotion Research Group, University of Oxford. www.heartstats. org.

Warnes CA, Liberthson R, Danielson GK, *et al.* (2001) Task force: 1. The changing profile of congenital heart disease in adult life. *Journal of the American College of Cardiology,* **37**, 1170–1175.

Wren C & O'Sullivan JJ (2001) Survival with congenital heart disease and need for follow up in adult life. *Heart,* **85**(4), 438–443.

CHAPTER 2

Services for the Adult with Congenital Heart Disease

Brief history of the specialty

Adult congenital heart disease is a fast-growing cardiovascular specialty reflecting largely the successes of pediatric cardiology and cardiac surgery programs. Over 50% of infants would have died before reaching adulthood, had it not been for early surgical intervention. Prospects were far poorer for most patients with congenital heart disease until the second half of the 20th century.

'Modern' cardiology was born at the turn of the 19th century with the development of radiography (Roentgen, 1895) and electrocardiography (Einthoven, 1903). The first therapeutic milestones for congenital heart disease came with Robert Gross in Boston (ligation of a patent arterial duct, 1939), Clarence Crafoord in Stockholm (resection of aortic coarctation, 1944), and Alfred Blalock and Helen Taussig in Baltimore (the shunt operation for palliation of cyanosed patients with congenital heart disease, 1944).

Until the 1940s, congenital heart disease was understood primarily from autopsy information. The 1947 publication of *Congenital Malformations of the Heart* by Helen Taussig illuminated the clinical perspective of the story, by making the malformations of the heart understandable and accessible.

The child with congenital heart disease was previously coddled and activities were restricted. Taussig strongly opposed this view: 'The two most important considerations in the care of patients with congenital malformations of the heart are: (1) allow the individual to lead as normal a life as possible and (2) surround him with an atmosphere of confidence expectation that will grow.'

In 1953, John Gibbon in Philadelphia performed the first successful operation employing a mechanical heart/lung bypass system for closure of an atrial septal defect. Walton Lillehei and Richard Varco in 1954 performed the first successful repair of tetralogy of Fallot—with the aid of controlled cross-circulation with another human as a pump-oxygenator—at the University of Minnesota. In 1955, John W. Kirklin at the Mayo Clinic reported eight cases of intracardiac surgery using the Gibbon type mechanical pump-oxygenator. Donald Ross in 1966 in London, England, used for the first time aortic homografts (human valves) to repair tetralogy of Fallot with pulmonary atresia, and soon after to complete the pulmonary autograft procedure for aortic valve disease (an operation that carries his name). Further major surgical advances were the arterial switch procedure for transposition of great arteries (Jatene, 1976), the introduction of the Fontan concept (bypassing the right heart in patients with hypoplastic ventricles, where a biventricular circulation is not possible, Fontan, 1971) and the rationale for normalizing pulmonary and systemic blood flow early in life by repairing defects in infancy, introduced and popularized by Drs Yacoub and Castaneda in the 1970s (from London and Boston, respectively).

Other major breakthroughs such as the development of echocardiography, the use of prostaglandins, the introduction of catheter interventions (starting with Rashkind's balloon creation of an atrial septal defect as a palliation for patients with transposition of the great arteries in 1966) and more recently cardiac magnetic resonance imaging have all revolutionized the field. Surgical mortality, initially high even for simple lesions (20–30%), has fallen over the years and is currently well down to single figures, including operations for complex congenital heart disease.

Immense technical resources are now at our disposal, allowing for precise anatomic and physiologic diagnoses, with high levels of perioperative care, advanced aids of myocardial protection and an astonishing armament of palliative and reparative surgical and catheter procedures all being available for patients with congenital heart disease (CHD) in many places around the world.

Survival after pediatric cardiac surgery

Specific diagnostic categories are compared to a reference healthy population (Fig. 2.1).

While this is a dramatic success story of modern medicine, it has created a new population of patients who have not been cured. It is only recently that it has been appreciated that most ACHD patients have undergone reparative and not corrective surgery. Many of them face the prospect of further surgery, arrhythmias and heart failure and many are at increased risk of premature death. Furthermore, some patients with congenital lesions present late during adulthood. Most of these patients will, again, require and benefit from expert cardiology care.

Service provision

Care of the adult with congenital heart disease requires knowledge of the morphologic substrate, the type of surgical intervention employed, the postoperative cardiac and non-cardiac sequelae, and the acquired cardiac disease that accrues with age. Regional specialized comprehensive care facilities have evolved to address the needs of this complex and growing patient population around the world. These facilities do not compete with practicing physicians or community hospitals, but instead offer services difficult or impossible to duplicate elsewhere.

Attendance at a tertiary adult congenital cardiac center should be considered for:
1 the initial assessment of suspected or known congenital lesions;

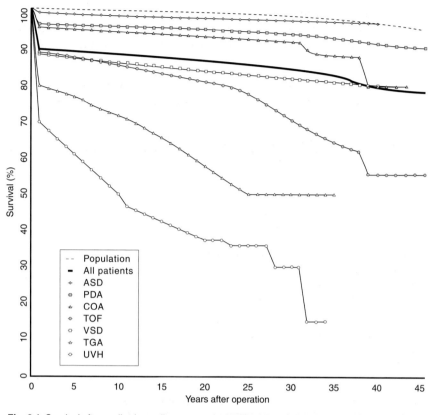

Fig. 2.1 Survival after pediatric cardiac surgery in the Finnish population study of patients with congenital heart disease. Specific diagnostic categories are compared to a reference healthy population. ASD, atrial septal defect; PDA, patent ductus arteriosus; COA, coarctation of the aorta; VSD, ventricular septal defect; TOF, tetralogy of Fallot; TGA, transposition of great arteries; UVH, univentricular heart. (With permission from Nieminen *et al.* (2001) *Circulation*, **104**: 573.)

2 follow-up and continuing care of patients with moderate and severe complex lesions;
3 further surgical and catheter intervention;
4 risk assessment and support for non-cardiac surgery and pregnancy.

However, the majority of adults with congenital heart disease will still require local follow-up for geographic, social, and health economic reasons. Primary care physicians and general adult cardiologists must, therefore, have some understanding of the health needs and special issues in the general medical management of this population. Importantly, community and hospital physicians must recognize when to promptly refer these patients to an expert center. Published management guidelines may assist in this process.

Organization of care
Care of the adult with congenital heart disease should be coordinated by

regional or national centers. Approximately one expert center should be created to serve a population of 5–10 million people. Satellite centers, with outpatient-based specialized services, may be encouraged to form direct links with the regional center.

- Adults with moderate and severe CHD (Table 2.1) will require periodic evaluation at a regional adult CHD center. These patients, as indeed all patients with

Table 2.1 Types of patients who should be seen at regional adult CHD centers

Absent pulmonary valve syndrome
Aorto-pulmonary window
Atrioventricular septal defects
Coarctation of the aorta
Common arterial trunk (or truncus arteriosus)
Congenitally corrected transposition of the great arteries
Cor triatriatum
Coronary artery anomalies (except incidental findings)
Criss-cross heart
Cyanotic congenital heart patients (all)
Double outlet ventricle
Double inlet ventricle
Ebstein anomaly
Eisenmenger syndrome
Fontan procedure
Interrupted aortic arch
Isomerism (heterotaxy syndromes)
Kawasaki's disease
Infundibular right ventricular outflow obstruction (moderate to severe)
Marfan syndrome (unless already established under expert leadership)
Mitral atresia
Partial or total anomalous pulmonary venous connection
Patent ductus arteriosus (not closed)
Pulmonary atresia (all forms)
Pulmonary hypertension complicating CHD
Pulmonary valve regurgitation (moderate to severe)
Pulmonary valve stenosis (moderate to severe)
Single ventricle
Sinus of Valsalva fistula/aneurysm
Subvalvar or supravalvar aortic stenosis
Tetralogy of Fallot
Transposition of the great arteries
Tricuspid atresia
Valved conduits
Vascular rings
Ventricular septal defects with: aortic regurgitation, coarctation, history of endocarditis, mitral valve disease, right ventricular outflow tract obstruction, straddling tricuspid and/or mitral valve, subaortic stenosis

Modified from Therrien J. *et al.* (2001) CCS Consensus Conference 2001 update: recommendations for the management of adults with congenital heart disease. *Canadian Journal of Cardiology,* **17**, 940–959, 1029–1050, and 1135–1158 (with permission).

CHD, should also have regular contact with their primary care physician (in a joint care model).

• Existing pediatric cardiology programs should identify an adult CHD center to which transfer of care should be made when patients reach adult age.

• Adult cardiology and cardiac surgical centers should have a referral relationship with a regional adult CHD center.

• Emergency care facilities should have an affiliation with a regional adult CHD center.

• Physicians without specific training and expertise in adult CHD should not manage adults with moderate and severe CHD independently, but in collaboration with colleagues with advanced training and experience in the care of such patients.

• Patients with moderate or severe CHD may require admission or transfer to a regional adult CHD center for urgent or acute care.

• Most cardiac catheterization and electrophysiologic procedures for adults with moderate and severe CHD should be performed at the regional center, where appropriate personnel and equipment are available. If such procedures are planned at the local cardiac center, prior consultation with adult CHD cardiology colleagues should be sought to avoid unnecessary duplication of invasive procedures.

• Cardiovascular surgical procedures in adults with moderate and severe CHD should generally be performed in a regional adult CHD center with specific experience in the surgical care of these patients.

• Appropriate links should be made for provision of care during pregnancy and for non-cardiac surgery. The need to develop an integrated team of high-risk obstetricians, anesthetists and adult CHD cardiologists cannot be overstated.

• Each regional center should develop a joint medical and surgical database, to record activity and outcomes, audit results and facilitate research. Comprehensive patient records should be kept in the regional adult CHD center and copied to the primary care physician and to the individual patient.

Manpower, training and research

The American College of Cardiology Task Force states that a minimum of two years of full-time ACHD training is needed for a senior cardiology trainee (with an adult or pediatric cardiology background) to become clinically competent, to contribute academically, and to effectively train others. Training programs for other key staff (e.g. nurses, obstetricians, imaging staff, technicians, psychologists) in adult CHD teams should also be established.

National and international curricula in adult CHD are held regularly to disseminate existing information on the management of the adult with CHD and stimulate research. Educational material is available to guide both patients and physicians. Barriers to multidisciplinary services should be challenged, with the objective of making expert resources available for all adult patients with CHD who need them.

There is a pressing need for clinical research on potential factors influencing the late outcome of this population. The effects of medical, catheter and surgical intervention need to undergo further prospective assessment. Clinical and research resources must, therefore, be secured for this large patient population.

Transition of care
Structural plans for transition from pediatric to adult CHD care need to be developed. Different models will apply depending on local circumstances. Collaboration between different disciplines is the key element to any transition program. Individual patient education regarding their diagnosis and specific health behaviors is part of this process and should start early. Patients and their families need to appreciate early the need for and merits of lifelong follow-up for their condition, and that further intervention including surgery may be required. Comprehensive information including diagnosis, previous surgical and or catheter interventions, medical therapy, investigations, current outpatient clinic reports and medication should be kept by the patient and also be sent to the adult CHD facility. The development of a patient electronic health 'passport' is to be encouraged for all patients and is absolutely essential for patients with complex CHD and numerous previous interventions.

The multiple needs of this population can be best fulfilled through national networks with the following objectives:
- to establish a network of regional centers;
- to foster professional specialist training;
- to coordinate national or local registries;
- to facilitate research.

Effective communication between units
Within this framework of patient care, general cardiologists with an interest need to be supported locally in district hospitals and be facilitated to work with both tertiary and primary care physicians to provide for the adult with CHD. Pediatric cardiology expertise must be utilized and transition care programs developed to ensure seamless care for CHD patients. Patients, and their families, need to realize that lifelong follow-up is required for most of them and that they may well require further intervention, medical and/or surgical, preferably before overt symptoms develop. Databases shared amongst pediatric, adult and non-tertiary care centers and easy access to regional facilities should be in place to promote this multilevel collaboration. Clinic records need to be communicated to all disciplines involved and copied to patients, who themselves should be encouraged to create their own health records. Patient advocacy groups need to continue to develop and participate actively in increasing general awareness of adult CHD issues and lobbying for and securing additional resources for clinical and research purposes.

Patient support groups

There are numerous patient self-help and awareness groups that both patients and physicians should be aware of and utilize.

- **GUCH**: Grown-Up Congenital Heart; term introduced by Dr Jane Somerville, one of the founders of the field. The Grown-Up Congenital Heart Patients Association (GUCH) is a UK charity, founded in 1993 to provide information and support for young people and adults who were born with a heart condition, and their families. www.guch.org
- **CACHNET.ORG (Canada)**. CACHNET.ORG is home to the Canadian Adult Congenital Heart Network and the Toronto Congenital Cardiac Centre For Adults at the University of Toronto. Their aim is to provide comprehensive care and information to adult patients with congenital heart disease and their care providers. www.cachnet.org
- **Adult Congenital Heart Association (US)**. The Adult Congenital Heart Association (ACHA) is an international organization that provides information and support for patients, their families and healthcare professionals. www.achaheart.org
- **Children's Heart Society**. At this site you will find information on the Society and resources for parents, family and children. www.childrensheart.org
- **National Marfan Foundation (US)**. The National Marfan Foundation was founded in 1981 by people who have the Marfan syndrome and their families. www.marfan.org
- **Noonan Syndrome Support Group (US)**. The group is intended for people whose lives are touched by Noonan syndrome. www.noonansyndrome.org
- **Down Syndrome Association (UK)**. The Down Syndrome Association exists to support people with Down syndrome, their family and carers, as well as providing information for those with a professional interest. The association also aims to improve general understanding and awareness of the condition and to champion the rights of people with Down syndrome. www.dsa-uk.com
- **Congenital Heart Defects.com**. This site is devoted to providing information to members of the worldwide congenital heart defect (CHD) community. www.congenitalheartdefects.com
- **The Congenital Heart Disease Resource Page**. Provides a collection of resources, including books, web resources, support groups and defect information. www.csun.edu/~hcmth011/heart
- **Children's Heart Information Network**. CHIN is an international organization that provides reliable information, support services and resources to families of children with congenital heart defects and acquired heart disease, adults with congenital heart defects, and the professionals who work with them. www.tchin.org
- **Pulmonary Hypertension Association (UK)**. The main aims of the PHA are to provide support, fellowship and educational resources for patients with pulmonary hypertension, their families, friends and members of the nursing and medical profession involved in the provision of their care. www.pha-uk.com

Professional and other useful websites

Numerous websites provide useful information on adult CHD exclusively or as part of a cardiology forum.

• ISACCD: International Society for Adult Congenital Cardiac Disease; ISACCD seeks to promote, maintain and pursue excellence in the care of adolescents and adults with congenital cardiac disease. The Society is dedicated to the advancement of knowledge and training in medical disciplines pertinent to congenital heart disease in adults. www.isaccd.org

• European Society of Cardiology (ESC) and the ESC Grown-up Congenital Heart Disease. www.escardio.org/society/wg/wg22.htm

• The Association for European Paediatric Cardiology. www.aepc.org/home. htm

• British Cardiac Society. www.bcs.com/

• British Heart Foundation. www.bhf.org.uk

• American College of Cardiology. www.acc.org

• American Heart Association. www.americanheart.org

• Canadian Adult Congenital Heart Network. www.cachnet.org

• Royal Brompton Adult Congenital Heart Unit. www.rbh.nthames.nhs.uk

• Japanese Society for Adult Congenital Heart Disease. www.jsachd.org

• Congenital Heart Surgeon's Society. www.chssdc.org

• 2000 Canadian Cardiovascular Society Consensus Conference on Adult Congenital Heart Disease. www.rbh.nthames.nhs.uk/Cardiology/Consensus/index.htm

• Proceedings of the 32nd Bethesda Conference Care of the Adult with Congenital Heart Disease. *Journal of the American College of Cardiology* 2001; **37**: 1161–1198. www.acc.org/clinical/bethesda/beth32/dirindex.htm

Further reading

Brickner ME, Hillis LD & Lange RA (2000) Congenital heart disease in adults. *New England Journal of Medicine*, **342**, 334–342.

Gatzoulis MA, Balaji S, Webber SA, *et al.* (2000) Risk factors for arrhythmia and sudden death in repaired tetralogy of Fallot: a multi-centre study. *Lancet*, **356**, 975–981.

Nieminen HP, Jokinen EV & Sairanen HI (2001) Late results of pediatric cardiac surgery in Finland: a population based study with 96% follow-up. *Circulation*, **104**, 570–575.

Therrien J *et al.* (2001) CCS Consensus Conference 2001 update: recommendations for the management of adults with congenital heart disease. *Canadian Journal of Cardiology*, **17**, 940–59, 1029–1050, and 1135–1158.

Webb GD, Williams RG, *et al.* (2001) 32nd Bethesda Conference: Care of the adult with congenital heart disease. *Journal of the American College of Cardiology*, **37**, 1161–1198.

CHAPTER 3

Pregnancy and Contraception

Professor Philip J. Steer
Academic Department of Obstetrics and Gynaecology, Chelsea and
Westminster Hospital & Faculty of Medicine, Imperial College, London, UK

Introduction

In the UK, the incidence of heart disease in pregnancy has declined during
the last half-century from about 3% to less than 1%. This has been due to the
dramatic reduction in the incidence of rheumatic fever following the introduction of penicillin (although rheumatic defects are still common in women
born overseas). However, about 0.8% of babies born have a congenital cardiac
anomaly, making this one of the largest groups of congenital defects. Because
of the improving results of surgical intervention over the last 30 years, more
now survive into the reproductive age group.

Current incidence of heart disease in pregnant women in the UK:
- Congenital   0.8%
- Acquired   0.1%

In the last UK confidential enquiry into maternal death (Lewis & Drife, 2004),
cardiac disease was the leading cause of maternal death after suicide. Moreover, the incidence is rising, with 44 deaths associated with cardiac disease in
the triennium 2000–2002 inclusive (up from 18 in 1988–1990), compared with
30 associated with thrombosis (33 in 1988–1990), 14 associated with hypertension (27 in 1988–1990) and 17 associated with hemorrhage (22 in 1988–1990).

Pre-conception counseling

More than 80% of women with congenital heart disease know about their treatment, occupational choices, and dental hygiene (Moons et al., 2001). Most have
some idea of the risks of pregnancy, but these are often inaccurate, ranging from
the unduly pessimistic to the inappropriately optimistic. Women approaching
reproductive age (from 12 years onwards) should be effectively counseled about
contraception, so that any pregnancies can be planned appropriately. Before becoming pregnant, they should receive detailed and tailored information about
the risks to them and their babies. Counseling should be set in motion by the
lead clinician involved in their care, which will usually be the cardiologist and
should involve an obstetrician/gynecologist with relevant experience. It is important that prior to conception a thorough and up-to-date understanding of the
woman's cardiologic status is made available and shared between all professionals involved and the patient and her partner. Therefore, as many investigations
as possible should be completed before pregnancy, so as to achieve this goal.

The cardiologist should discuss with each woman not only the effects of her heart disease on pregnancy, but also the effects of pregnancy on her heart disease.

Life expectancy

This is important because the woman may become unwell during her baby's childhood, and the need for family support during such a stressful time should be discussed. The issue of potential mortality both during pregnancy, and following the birth, should be addressed directly. Moreover, from the medicolegal perspective, it is important to give the woman some statistical estimate of the likelihood of mortality. This should be documented in the notes, and also communicated to the woman and her general practitioner in writing. Sending the woman a copy of a clearly written letter to the general practitioner is a useful way of doing this.

To put matters into context, it can be helpful to quote comparisons with the maternal mortality in the United Kingdom in the 1920s, which was one in 250. This is the same as India in the present day. In some parts of the developing world, the lifetime risk of dying from pregnancy can be as high as one in 10. Quoting these risks helps the woman to put her risk into perspective. It is important to make it clear to the woman that the risk of pregnancy is just that, a risk. Half the women with a 50% risk will survive pregnancy, but one in 1000 women with a 'low risk' will not. (See Table 3.1.)

It is not possible to give a list of lesions with precise risks attached, because few women have exactly the same lesion, and the risk is also strongly modulated by complications that may or may not develop during pregnancy. For this reason, there is no substitute for a careful appraisal of the facts for each individual, made jointly by the cardiologist and an obstetrician.

However, conditions in which risk of maternal death is likely to exceed 1% include:
- any form of cyanotic congenital heart disease;
- pulmonary hypertension;
- poor systemic ventricular function (for example, a systemic RV);
- severe left heart obstructive lesions (for example, mitral and aortic stenosis);
- Marfan disease, especially if the aortic root is dilated;
- women who have had a repair of coarctation with a Dacron patch;
- previous peripartum cardiomyopathy;
- poor cardiac function for any reason at the time of conception.

Table 3.1 Approximate risks of mortality associated with pregnancy

An entirely healthy woman	1 in 20,000
Average for the population	1 in 10,000
Corrected Fallot's or similar	1 in 1,000
Severe aortic stenosis	1 in 100
Pulmonary hypertension	1 in 3
Eisenmenger's complex	1 in 2

Risks to the fetus
Intrauterine growth restriction
Women with cyanotic congenital heart disease often have to be delivered early because of poor fetal growth (up to 50% risk of intrauterine growth restriction).

Fetal abnormality
Women with congenital heart lesions should be advised that their children are likely to be at increased risk of a similar defect. It has been traditional to quote a figure for recurrence of approximately 3–5%, but there is increasing evidence that the risk varies according to the maternal defect (see Table 3.2), for example:

Women with mechanical heart valves requiring warfarin therapy experience a high rate of fetal loss, from warfarin embryopathy in the first trimester, to intracranial hemorrhage from fetal anticoagulation in the middle trimester (Romano-Zelekha *et al.*, 2001).

The issue of the possibility of termination of pregnancy if the fetus is found to have a severe lesion should be explained and discussed.

In some women, the desire for pregnancy may be an important indication for expediting surgery, if this is likely to be necessary at some time anyway. For example, the risk of death or major complications associated with pregnancy in a woman with uncorrected Fallot's tetralogy may be as high as 10%, but falls dramatically for most patients who have undergone corrective surgery.

An important issue is that of *patient autonomy*. It has been traditional in the past to talk about 'allowing women with heart disease to become pregnant', or 'telling women with heart disease that they must not become pregnant'. Current best practice is to treat the patient wherever possible as a partner in the management of their condition, eschewing a paternalistic (or maternalistic) approach. Rather, one should explore sympathetically a woman's natural desire to have children and help her to work through the implications of this for herself, the children, her partner and their families. One should encourage the woman to make her own decision about her personal priorities, and then

Maternal abnormality	Recurrence risk (%)
Marfans syndrome	50
Ventricular septal defect	15
Atrial septal defect	10
Aortic stenosis	10
Tetralogy of Fallot*	3

Table 3.2 Recurrence risks of maternal abnormalities

*Assuming the mother is negative for the DiGeorge microdeletion mutation. The full 22q11 deletion has a dominant inheritance and causes a variety of phenotypes plus metabolic defects secondary to hypoplasia of the parathyroid and thymus glands.

support her in the decision. It is particularly for this reason that one must not obfuscate the risk of death, as otherwise one can be accused of encouraging pregnancy in women who are not fully aware of the risks.

Finally, the need for detailed and time-consuming antenatal care should be emphasized. Maternal cardiac disease is one of the few remaining valid indications for hospital admission for bed rest. Because many women live some distance from the nearest maternity/cardiac center, they may need to reside in the hospital for medical or social reasons for anything from 4 weeks to 4 months in the latter stages of pregnancy.

The effects of pregnancy on the cardiovascular system

Pregnancy is an additional stress on an already compromised cardiovascular system. There is a 50% expansion in blood volume, mostly due to retention of fluid and relative enlargement of the plasma volume, which is necessary to provide appropriate blood flow to the uterus and fetoplacental unit. This increase in volume is associated with:

• an increase in heart rate from as early as 6 weeks' gestation;
• peripheral vasodilatation to allow for increased blood flow and heat loss (heat is generated by the growing fetus);
• a fall in systemic venous resistance;
• a 50% increase in cardiac output.

Women who just manage to cope in the non-pregnant state may experience cardiac decompensation during pregnancy. On the other hand, if the increase in cardiac output is limited, fetal growth may be adversely affected. Changes in peripheral vascular resistance often lead to changes in left-to-right and right-to-left shunting. The aortic dilatation associated with increased cardiac output increases the risk of aortic rupture in women with repaired coarctation, bicuspid aortic valve aortopathy and in Marfan syndrome.

Another major issue is the activation of the coagulation system that occurs during pregnancy, probably as an adaptation to limit postpartum hemorrhage. Pregnant women are five times more likely to have a thrombotic episode than non-pregnant women, and this likelihood is further increased if the woman has a high hemoglobin concentration, such as occurs in cyanotic heart disease.

Another major cardiovascular threat that can occur even in normal pregnancy is the development of pre-eclampsia. Although there is a moderate fall in blood pressure in the middle trimester, blood pressure usually rises again towards term. In 12–15% of women, this rise is marked (pregnancy-induced hypertension). In 2–3% of women, multisystem disorder accompanies this hypertension, and when significant proteinuria develops, the woman is diagnosed as having pre-eclampsia. However, more important than the renal dysfunction is the clotting abnormality (diffuse intravascular coagulation) that complicates a significant proportion of cases. More rarely there is liver and cerebral involvement, both of which can be fatal. The combination of pre-eclampsia and Eisenmenger's syndrome is usually fatal.

Other increased risks in pregnancy include:

- infection (for example urinary tract infection);
- increased risk of subacute bacterial endocarditis;
- hemorrhage (both antepartum and postpartum hemorrhage pose particular risks for women with limited cardiac reserve);
- arrhythmia (myocardial excitability is increased during pregnancy).

Antenatal care

Care of this high-risk group of pregnant women should be provided by fully trained personnel, preferably at consultant level. Moreover, such consultants should have experience or training in pregnancy in women with cardiac disease, who are best looked after in a specialist unit. Regular visits will need to be more frequent than in women with a normal pregnancy (for example, every 2 weeks until 24 weeks and then weekly), and a much more thorough examination should be carried out at each visit than is necessary in women without medical complications. It is probably good practice at each visit to:
- measure the pulse rate and blood pressure
- assess the heart rhythm
- auscultate the heart sounds
- listen to the lung bases.

Such a thorough examination can pick up the early signs of pathology developing, such as:
- ventricular decompensation (results in a tachycardia)
- onset of arrhythmia
- the development of bacterial endocarditis
- incipient pulmonary edema.

Prompt management before major decompensation occurs can prevent many problems. At each visit, the woman should be asked specifically about any shortness of breath or palpitations. Antenatal records which we have designed specifically for the care of women with cardiac disease during pregnancy are illustrated in Fig. 3.1. Periodic echocardiography and other imaging should be individualized according to patients' specific cardiovascular status. Typically, close monitoring is required for patients with evidence of deteriorating cardiac function, the appearance of a new murmur, or those at risk of silent deterioration (for example, aortic root dilatation in Marfan syndrome).

Because of the increased risk of congenital heart disease in the fetus, it is essential to offer the woman appropriate screening ultrasound scans. These are listed below.

Fetal nuchal translucency measurement at 12–13 weeks

This involves the measurement of the nuchal skinfold thickness at the back of the fetal neck. The normal thickness is less than 4 mm. The thickness, taken in conjunction with a woman's age (and increasingly, with other biochemical measurements such as beta HCG) has about 85% sensitivity for Down syndrome (which is itself associated with cardiac defects). Studies have also

PREGNANCY PLAN

Name:

Cardiac lesion:

Delivery plan:

S/B Cardiologist:

EDD:

S/B Anesthetist:

Maternal echocardiogram at:

Treatment at booking:

Fetal anomaly scan:

Fetal echocardiogram:

	weeks
Plan	
Ordered	
Result	

Date	Ges-tation	SOB	Palpi-tations	Other symptoms	BP	Pulse rate	Pulse rhythm	Murmur	Lung bases	Edema	SFH	Present-ation	5ths palp	FH	Urine	Current treatment	Hb	Next appointment	Signature

Fig. 3.1 Antenatal records for women with cardiac disease. Courtesy of High Risk Obstetric Team, Chelsea & Westminster Hospital, London, UK.

shown that congenital heart disease per se is associated with about a 60% chance of an increased nuchal thickness (>95th centile), although the positive predictive value of an increased nuchal thickness for cardiac disease is not very high (1.5%) (Hyett *et al.*, 1999). However, the incidence of congenital cardiac disease if the nuchal thickness is normal is only one in 1,000, so it is useful for reassuring mothers at increased risk because they have congenital heart disease themselves. In addition, improving ultrasound resolution has enabled the direct detection of structural lesions even at this early gestation, so that detection rates of up to 90% have been reported (Carvalho, 2001).

Fetal echocardiography at 14–16 weeks
This is offered if there is a particularly strong history of congenital heart disease. It allows early detection of moderate to severe lesions, but because the fetal heart is still very small at this gestation, additional echocardiography later is necessary.

Routine fetal anomaly scan at 20 weeks
Most women in the UK are now offered a routine screening fetal anomaly scan at about 20 weeks' gestation. This includes a four-chamber view of the fetal heart, which has been shown to detect up to 80% of major cardiac lesions.

Fetal echocardiography at 18–22 weeks
Because of the increased risk attached to mothers with congenital heart disease, it is important that a scan is carried out by a trained fetal cardiologist in addition to the routine anomaly scan. The structures are easier to make out at 18–22 weeks' gestation. If there remains any doubt, additional scans at 24 or even 26 weeks may be necessary. It is also good practice for the baby of the mother with congenital heart disease to be examined carefully following birth and before discharge from hospital, as some lesions can only be detected once the ductus arteriosus and the physiological atrial septal defect closes following birth. A postnatal echocardiogram is only necessary if a clinical abnormality is found.

Fetal surveillance
In women with good hemodynamic function and normal oxygen saturations, there is no evidence that routine ultrasound surveillance of fetal growth is necessary. Indeed, excessively frequent scans may increase maternal anxiety, and can lead to over-intervention, such as unnecessary induction of labor. Instead, ultrasound scans for fetal growth should be ordered when specifically indicated. Indications include increased hemoglobin concentrations in the mother (reduces placental perfusion), restrictive lesions where cardiac output is limited, women who are underweight or markedly hypo- or hypertensive, and women with a previous history of intrauterine growth restriction. Clinical monitoring of fetal growth is carried out using symphysio-fundal height measurements, and scans should also be ordered if clinical growth is unsatisfactory.

Other aspects of care

Joint clinics between the obstetrician, cardiologist and anesthetist are an essential component of good management. They enable careful planning of pregnancy care, and in particular, discussion of labor and delivery.

It is also important that women have access to experienced midwives during their antenatal care, because the majority of these women will have a relatively normal labor and delivery, for which they will need supervision from an experienced midwife with appropriate high dependency skills. In addition, they need instruction in how to deal with labor and care for their newborn baby. In many European countries, the midwife is the expert in these areas of care.

Risks related to specific cardiac conditions

For more information on risks, see Further reading: Task Force on the Management of Cardiovascular Diseases During Pregnancy of the European Society of Cardiology (2003).

Tetralogy of Fallot

The main risk in patients with unrepaired tetralogy is related to the degree of maternal cyanosis. When the oxygen saturation falls below 85%, further desaturation can interfere with fetal oxygenation, leading either to fetal growth restriction or even intrauterine death. Close monitoring of blood pressure and oxygen saturations is needed, and vasodilators should be avoided because they increase the right-to-left shunt.

Coarctation of the aorta

Most women with this condition will have been diagnosed before pregnancy, and the repair will have been carried out. However, aneurysm formation at the site of the repair, or even rupture of the aorta, can occur and such complications are reported in about 1% of cases. In addition, even following repair, some women are left with a persistent hypertension which is difficult to control. Restriction of physical activity should be recommended to avoid surges in blood pressure, and clinical management should also be directed at avoiding high blood pressure. In this context, pre-eclampsia presents a particular risk.

Transposition of the great arteries

In most women born in the last 25 years, this will have been anatomically corrected by the 'switch' operation and the residual risk will be small. However, physiologic correction using 'atrial baffles' like the Mustard procedure leaves some women with impaired systemic ventricular function and a substantially increased risk of thrombotic complications secondary to impaired flow. Use of subcutaneous low-molecular-weight heparin should be considered.

Congenitally corrected transposition of the great arteries

The main problem here is that the systemic right ventricle may fail under the additional strain of pregnancy. Again, stress limitation is important. If the patient shows any signs of developing right ventricular decompensation, early delivery is recommended.

Marfan syndrome

Marfan syndrome is relatively common, with an incidence of one in 5000 women. There is deficient elastic tissue in the blood vessels due to a dominantly inherited fibrillin-1 deficiency disorder. The major risk is of aortic root dilatation, producing either aortic incompetence, or even more seriously, dissection of the aorta. The risk of death or serious morbidity is probably about 1% when the aortic root is less than 4 cm in diameter, but increases to as much as 10% as the diameter of the root increases. Although successful pregnancies have been reported with aortic root diameters as large as 7.9 cm, the risk is reduced if such dilated roots are electively replaced with Dacron grafts before pregnancy. Similar problems can occur in women with the Ehlers-Danlos syndrome or bicuspid aortic valves.

Mitral stenosis

This is the main lesion seen in women who have had rheumatic fever. The normal area of the mitral valve is about 4–6 cm^2. Below an area of 1.5 cm^2 there is a risk that blood cannot pass through the valve at an adequate rate at times of stress, leading to the development of pulmonary edema, congestive heart failure and intrauterine growth restriction. In the past, closed valvotomy was used if symptoms or signs developed, but more recently percutaneous balloon mitral valvotomy has been used successfully.

Aortic stenosis

Less common than mitral stenosis, aortic stenosis can lead to similar problems, and as with left ventricular inflow stenosis, restriction of activity and avoidance of increasing output requirements are key to management. Occasionally, patients with evidence of early left ventricular decompensation require relief of aortic stenosis with either catheter balloon valvuloplasty or cardiac surgery.

Pregnancy in women with heart valve prostheses

The problem in managing such women is balancing the risk to the mother with the risk to the fetus. In most cases, the hemodynamic performance of the heart is good. The main risk is of valve thrombosis. For this reason, most women are anticoagulated with warfarin. This drug is very effective at preventing valve thrombosis, but unfortunately it crosses the placenta. This can lead to warfarin embryopathy in up to 80% of fetuses. In addition, because the fetus is also anticoagulated, 70% of pregnancies have a poor fetal outcome, with increased incidence of middle trimester miscarriage, internal fetal bleeding, and central nervous system fetal abnormalities. The latter can be due to cerebral intraventricular hemorrhage and resultant hydrocephalus. For many years, the usual recommendation has been to change the women on to intravenous heparin for the first trimester. This appears to be effective at preventing valve thrombosis, but carries long-term problems of bone demineralization, maternal bleeding, and infection from the venous access sites required. For this reason, most authorities have recommended recommencing warfarin at 12 weeks' gestation, reverting to intravenous heparin from 36 weeks, and stopping the heparin temporarily during the time of delivery. Following this, the warfarin is restarted (it is safe in breastfeeding mothers as very little passes into the breast milk). Because of the high fetal loss rate with warfarin, subcutaneous low-molecular-weight heparin in the second and third trimester has been tried instead. Unfortunately, most reports suggest that valve clotting complications still occur (in about 10% of women). Thus, women are faced with a strategy which either minimizes the risk to themselves, or to their fetus, with currently no therapeutic approach which is safe for both.

Cardiomyopathy

It is important to distinguish between pre-existing cardiomyopathy not associated with pregnancy, and peripartum cardiomyopathy. The outcome for the former, whether it is dilated or hypertrophic, is good (with appropriate management). However, with peripartum cardiomyopathy, mortality rates between 6% and 50% have been reported. Systemic and pulmonary embolism from mural thrombosis, and dysrhythmias, are important complications. Failure of the heart to return to its normal size within 6 months is a poor prognostic indicator, and suggests that any future pregnancies will be high risk.

Pulmonary hypertension

At one time it was thought that secondary pulmonary hypertension might be less serious than the primary form. However, more recent reports suggest that both are very risky, with maternal mortality rates of 30–50%. Many of those afflicted have a shunt, which eventually leads to cyanosis. A key part of the management strategy is anticoagulant prophylaxis. Subcutaneous low-molecular-weight heparin seems effective and may even need to be at therapeutic levels in the puerperium, when the risk of thrombosis is highest. Continuous nasal oxygen at 3 to 5 liters per minute antenatally raises maternal oxygen saturation by about 5%, and experience suggests that it improves fetal growth. It may also prevent pulmonary hypertensive crises. Management of delivery should be absolutely pain-free. In severe cases inhaled nitric oxide or prostacyclin, or even intravenous prostacyclin, may play an additional role.

Arrhythmias

Arrhythmias can usually be managed in much the same way as in women who are not pregnant. All commonly used anti-arrhythmic drugs cross the placenta, but most (for example, adenosine and flecainide) appear to be relatively safe for the fetus. Exceptions include some beta-blockers such as sotalol or propranolol, which interfere with fetal growth and may prevent proper fetal response to stress during labor. Amiodarone can be used, but may produce neonatal thyroid dysfunction, and the neonate should be followed up carefully with thyroid function tests. Most reports of electrical cardioversion are reassuring, with only rare anecdotal evidence of any fetal side-effects.

Special investigations and procedures during pregnancy

With modern echocardiographic techniques, there is usually no need to perform fluoroscopic or invasive investigations during pregnancy. However, if these are needed, chest radiography carries a negligible risk for the fetus, especially if the fetus is shielded by a lead apron over the mother's abdomen during any procedures. Computerized tomography, however, involves a much higher dosage of x-rays, and should therefore be avoided. Magnetic resonance imaging is safe. Transesophageal echocardiography can be carried out also if necessary.

If surgical intervention is necessary, this should be done without cardiopulmonary bypass whenever possible, as this procedure carries a significant risk for the fetus. However, the major risk of fetal damage occurs with hypothermia, and as long as normothermia and good maternal oxygenation is maintained, the fetus is likely to survive even cardiopulmonary bypass successfully.

Labor and delivery

The place of cesarean section

It has been customary in the past to recommend elective cesarean section for many women with congenital heart disease. The rationale for this has been the ability to program timing of delivery and ensure the presence of senior experienced personnel. In fact, any service that provides care for women with heart disease must be able to provide a 24-hour 7 days a week service for all 52 weeks of the year, because pregnant women can present with complications, labor, or other emergencies, at any time of the day or night. Accordingly, great effort should be made to ensure a consistent standard of care 24 hours a day.

Ensuring the availability of high-quality care at all times means that it is unnecessary to recommend routine cesarean section (CS). Vaginal delivery carries about half the risk of an elective cesarean section. For example, even elective CS increases the risks of hemorrhage twofold, clotting threefold and infection tenfold. While it is true that emergency cesarean sections can be particularly dangerous, and they are prevented by elective CS, detailed supervision during labor can reduce the incidence of unexpected emergencies to a low level. Under these circumstances, the risk of an intrapartum CS will be closer to that of an elective CS.

The key principle is to manage the stress of labor so that it does not exceed the woman's capacity to cope with it. In this regard, epidural anesthesia has a major part to play. The development of the low-dose slow incremental epidural, with its minimal effects on hemodynamic performance, has proved to be an important advance in the care of pregnant women with heart disease.

Induction of labor

Spontaneous labor is quicker, and carries a higher chance of a successful vaginal delivery, than induced labor. Accordingly, induction of labor should be carried out only for the usual obstetric indications. The commonest of these will be post-dates pregnancy, and currently induction is recommended at 7 to 10 days after the due date. Exceptions are obviously the cases where cardiac decompensation is likely or actually occurring. For such patients, careful consideration should be given to elective CS. Another indication for elective CS is the possibility of a sudden onset of a decompensating arrhythmia.

First and second stages of labor

Uterine contractions have been suggested in themselves to increase cardiovascular stress. Our experience is that with effective epidural anesthesia they have no readily observable effect. On the other hand, maternal 'bearing down' in the second stage of labor is a high-risk time, as it calls for very intense effort on the part of the mother. Accordingly, an estimation of hemodynamic reserve should be made antenatally, and recommendations made as to how long the woman can reasonably bear down without undue risk. A time limit should be set, after which delivery should be assisted either by ventouse extraction, or by forceps.

The third stage of labor

Management of the third stage (delivery of placenta and membranes) is another high-risk time. This is because, with uterine retraction, there is a transfusion of extra blood (previously in the maternal placental bed) into the maternal circulation, which can cause circulatory overload. On the other hand, if retraction fails to occur effectively, uterine hemorrhage will begin, and this can destabilize the circulation in the opposite direction. Management should therefore aim to minimize these fluctuations. Oxytocic drugs which are routinely used in the third stage also have major hemodynamic effects. Ergometrine increases the blood pressure substantially in most women, whereas Syntocinon® reduces it. The combination often used (Syntometrine®) has unpredictable effects, which can go either way. Our practice has therefore been not to give bolus injections of these medications, but to start a continuous infusion of a low-dose rate of Syntocinon® (at about 10–12 mU min^{-1}), which at this dosage has minimal cardiovascular effects. It should be given in a low volume of fluid, so as not to overload the circulation with crystalloid. The infusion can be continued for 4 to 12 hours, depending on the circumstances. At the time of cesarean section, one can also use uterine compression sutures, thus avoiding the need for oxytocics altogether.

Monitoring in labor

Continuous fetal monitoring is recommended in all cases to ensure maximum surveillance of the fetus. Particular attention needs to be paid to patients on beta-blockers, as the latter may suppress signs of fetal distress. Maternal monitoring during labor should be individualized according to the mother's particular pathology, but is likely to include:

- continuous EKG monitoring;
- pulse oximetry;
- invasive blood pressure monitoring using an arterial line.

An arterial line in place is particularly useful if the mother's cardiac output falls substantially, as automated external blood pressure monitors and pulse oximetry often provide unreliable information when systemic hypotension with hemodynamic compromise are present.

Antibiotic prophylaxis

There is no evidence that routine antibiotic prophylaxis is necessary if the woman has a spontaneous vaginal delivery. It is probably wise, however, to give such prophylaxis (usually with penicillin and gentamicin) if the woman has any form of operative vaginal delivery, or a cesarean section. The repair of a small or moderate size episiotomy or tear does not require antibiotic prophylaxis, but if the tear is extensive, and particularly if it is third degree, then antibiotics should be given. They should also be given if the woman has previously had endocarditis or has artificial heart valves. (See Chapter 4 on infective endocarditis prophylaxis.)

We find it useful to have a ready prepared sheet outlining the clinical management plan for delivery (Fig. 3.2). It has on it ready prepared options which simply have to be ticked or circled in order to indicate the consensus about preferred management. This not only structures predelivery multidisciplinary discussion, but also acts as a useful aide memoire for the staff present at the delivery. A second sheet gives examples of common complications that arise, together with specific recommendations for dealing with them (Fig. 3.3).

The puerperium

The most important routine aspect of care in the puerperium is thromboprophylaxis. It is usual to give a prophylactic dose of subcutaneous low-molecular-weight heparin.

Another important aspect which is often overlooked is breastfeeding. Most of the medications used in cardiac women, such as digoxin, or flecainide, are safe during breastfeeding because insignificant amounts get into the breast milk. However, as some beta-blockers such as sotalol or propranolol can get into the breast milk in sufficient amounts to cause fetal bradycardia, either they should be avoided or the mother should be advised to breastfeed only with careful supervision of the baby to ensure that it is not being affected. The British National Formulary provides useful and authoritative information on this aspect of care. Involvement of the neonatologist is also important, especially if the baby is preterm or growth restricted.

Joint Cardiac Obstetric Service (JCOS) management plan for delivery

Cardiac diagnosis ....

Please circle agreed plan and tick box when actioned

If admitted to labor ward	**Please inform** Obstetrician on call Anesthetist on call Cardiac team	**Grade** **Consultant/registrar** **Consultant/registrar** **Y/N**	Tick
Antenatal admission	From .... weeks		
Mode of delivery	Elective lower cesarean section/trial of vaginal delivery		
Cesarean section	*3rd stage:* Prophylactic compression suture/Syntocinon 5 units over 10–20 mins/Syntocinon – low dose infusion (8–12 milliunits/min) *Anesthetic technique:* Epidural/spinal/general/other *Comments* .... *Maternal monitoring:* EKG/SaO$_2$/non-invasive BP/invasive BP/CVP *Other instructions/warnings:* .... **Inform JCOS member if admitted to labor before scheduled LSCS date**		
Vaginal delivery 1st stage	HDU chart/TEDS in labor/medication to be continued .... *Prophylactic antibiotics:* Elective/if operative delivery Epidural for analgesia: none/when requested/as soon as in established labor *Comments re anesthetic* .... Maternal monitoring: EKG/SaO$_2$/non-invasive BP/invasive BP/CVP		
Vaginal delivery 2nd stage	Normal second stage/short second stage (then assist if not del max .... mins pushing)/elective assisted delivery only		
Vaginal delivery 3rd stage	Normal active management (oxytocin and CCT)/Syntocinon infusion 8–12 milliunits/min Continue syntocinon infusion .... hours		
Post delivery	High Dependency Unit (min stay .... hrs)/LMW heparin (duration ....) Other drugs postpartum		

Please inform the consultant obstetrician on call if there is departure from planned management or if new clinical situations develop

Fig. 3.2 Delivery management plan for women with cardiac disease. Courtesy of High Risk Obstetric Team, Chelsea & Westminster Hospital, London, UK. EKG, electrocardiogram; SaO$_2$, oxygen saturations; BP, blood pressure; CVP, central venous pressure; HDU, high dependency unit; TEDS, thromboembolic deterrent stockings; CCT, controlled cord traction; LMW, low molecular weight.

Please inform the consultant obstetrician on call if there is departure from planned management or if clinical situations develop in women with cardiac disease

Examples of clinical situations	Consider the following
Spontaneous labor and recent thromboprophylaxis use eg LMWH/ Warfarm	Inform anesthetist ASAP Discuss with senior obstetric physicians Options may include ....
Need for Syntocinon augmentation in labor	• Use double strength Syntocinon but halve rate to reduce total volume of fluids given *(This decision needs to be taken at consultant level)*
Postpartum hemorrhage	• Inform anesthetic consultant on call • Consider use of compression suture • Consider use of intrauterine balloon (antibiotic cover is required) • Strict input/output charts to be maintained • Consider central access or arterial monitoring • Caution should be exercised in use of usual uterotonics eg misoprostol/hemabate/high dose Syntocinon infusion
Preterm labor	Do not use Ritrodrine or Salbutomol Atosiban (Tractocile) should be first line Mx
Pacemaker	Avoid bipolar diathermy and use unipolar
Useful contact details of JCOS team	

Please seek advice from JCOS member if there are concerns or if clarification is required on clinical management

Fig. 3.3 Examples of common complications during delivery and what to do. Courtesy of High Risk Obstetric Team, Chelsea & Westminster Hospital, London, UK. LMWH, low-molecular-weight heparin; Mx, management; JCOS, cardiac obstetric care service.

Contraception

The ideal contraceptive has not yet been invented; all methods have advantages and disadvantages. In women with heart disease, many of the side-effects of contraceptive techniques are increased or particularly important. On the other hand, unplanned and unwanted pregnancies almost invariably carry an even higher risk. Accordingly, some additional risks from use of the contraceptive may have to be accepted. The key features of contraception are reliability and safety.

Reliability

No method of contraception, even hysterectomy, is totally guaranteed to prevent pregnancy. Failure rates are measured as the PEARL index. This is the number of pregnancies that would occur if 100 women of average fertility used the method for 1 year. The average pregnancy rate if no contraception is used is 85 (about 15% of couples have a problem conceiving).

Safety

Women with heart disease are especially susceptible to those methods which increase the tendency of thrombosis. This is due in part to impaired circulation in the periphery, and in some women to an elevated hemoglobin concentration secondary to hypoxemia. In addition, if the heart is malformed it can cause sluggish blood flow that also increases the risks of clot formation and embolism. Another risk is infection. The roughened surfaces of the heart, valves or blood vessels can allow bacteria circulating in the blood to settle and cause endocarditis.

Methods available
'Natural methods'

There are a variety of techniques that use our understanding of how conception occurs to try and prevent pregnancy. Although often called 'natural', many seem far from natural in practice. For example, *abstinence* is completely effective but for many defeats the purpose of having a relationship!

Withdrawal (removing the penis before ejaculation) is not reliable because many men ejaculate a little sperm even before orgasm. Many couples intend to use it but at the vital moment prefer not to withdraw.

The so-called *'safe period'* relies on the assumption that the average woman ovulates 14 days from the beginning of her last menstrual period. Conception usually only occurs if intercourse takes place around the time of ovulation (sperm can survive for up to 72 hours and the egg for about 24 hours if not fertilized). Unfortunately, many women have irregular cycles and so they cannot rely on timing alone. In addition, recent studies suggest that some women may ovulate more than once during a single cycle. There are various devices for measuring temperature (the woman's temperature rises after ovulation due to secretion of progesterone from the developing corpus luteum) or the thickness of the mucus from the cervix (progesterone causes thickening of the cervical mucus). They can usually detect when ovulation has occurred, so if 48 hours is allowed, intercourse is unlikely to result in a pregnancy until after the next period. This means that love-making is only safe for about 10 days a month, and many couples find this irksome (it is sometimes known as the 'rhythm and blues' method). The reliability of these techniques is not very good (for example, a viral cold plays havoc with a temperature chart), and depends very much on how carefully they are used. They don't have any side-effects themselves, but tend to be associated with frustration and also with pregnancy! For women with high-risk lesions who cannot afford any risk of accidental pregnancy, such methods are inadequate.

Barrier methods

The commonest method is the male *sheath* or *condom*. It is quite effective, but sometimes condoms tear or slip off. They have to be used very carefully, and to make them really reliable, the woman has to insert a spermicide jelly into the vagina before intercourse. They are very safe, and have almost no side-effects (other than unwanted pregnancy, and the very rare problem of latex allergy), and also protect against sexually transmitted diseases. The failure rate ranges from 2% to 50%, depending on how carefully they are used.

Women can also use condoms made of polyurethane rather than latex or rubber. They are open at the outside end and closed at the inside end. Both ends have a flexible ring used to keep the condom in place. Among typical couples who use female condoms, about 21% will experience an accidental pregnancy in the first year. If these condoms are used consistently and correctly, about 5% will become pregnant. It is sometimes awkward to insert and it can make rustling noises during use, which puts some people off.

The *diaphragm* fits into the vagina, and lies between the introitus and the cervix, wedged between the posterior fornix and the symphysis pubis. It has to be used with a spermicide cream and inserted into the vagina before intercourse. It needs to be left in place for at least 6 hours after intercourse, until all the sperm have been killed. It requires some practice to use it effectively. It is not quite as effective as the condom in preventing pregnancy or infection.

The main problem for all these methods is the failure rate. If pregnancy occurs, termination may be the best option other than carrying on with the pregnancy. Many hormone changes occur in early pregnancy which make it quite stressful for the heart, and the anesthetics and procedures associated with termination of pregnancy are not without risk in women with severe heart disease. Termination of pregnancy is about half as dangerous as continuing with the pregnancy.

Coils or intrauterine contraceptive devices (IUCDs)

These are much more reliable than barrier methods. Some studies suggest that as few as one woman in 100 will get pregnant every 5 years of use (PEARL index 0.2). There are two main types; those wrapped in copper (e.g. *Saf-T-coil*) and those impregnated with a progestagen (hormone similar to progesterone) (e.g. the *Mirena* coil). Copper coils have been used for a long time and are widely available. Their main problems are that they can make periods heavy, and they can cause infection in the uterus, which can even spread to the fallopian tubes. For this reason, they are not suitable for nulliparous women (their uterus is much more susceptible to infection, for reasons that are not fully understood). Some cardiologists worry about the release of bacteria into the bloodstream, causing endocarditis, although the risk is probably very small. The most dangerous time is during insertion, and antibiotics should then be given as for dental work, except that a broader spectrum antibiotic is needed to deal with bacteria found in the vagina. In addition, although most intrauterine coils are inserted without anesthetic, they can occasionally cause a marked vagal bradycardia with hypotension. This can be dangerous in women with heart disease, and it is therefore recommended that any coil insertions are done in an operating theatre with appropriate anesthetic staff in attendance, in case a complication should occur. Mirena coils reduce menstrual bleeding rather than increasing it, and amenorrhea is common. They also cause much less infection than copper coils. A rare complication of all coils is ectopic pregnancy, but these are very rare with the Mirena coil. Many now consider this the contraceptive of choice for women with heart disease. They can be left in situ for up to 5 years at a time, and there are of course no problems with compliance. Expulsion rates are also very low.

Oral contraceptive pills

There are two main sorts, those with both estrogen and progestagen hormones (the *combined* pill), and those with only a very low dose of progestagen (the *low-dose* or *mini* pill). The *combined* pill is the most effective, with failure rates of less than one in 1000 women per year (PEARL index 0.1) if taken correctly—although studies show that up to a third of women find it difficult to remember to take their pill every day. It has many advantages, especially in regulating periods and reducing the amount of blood loss. However, the most important complication is that it can cause thrombosis. This risk is about three to four times higher in women taking the pill – up from one in 20,000 per year to about one in 5000 per year. In about a quarter of cases, the thrombosis is fatal. However, the risk for the average woman is still only about half that of dying from being pregnant. However, as long as the heart condition does not especially predispose to thrombosis, this may be a good choice because it is so effective.

By contrast, the low-dose or *progestagen-only* pill (POP) has almost no dangerous side-effects. It does not cause thrombosis. However, it has a failure rate considerably higher than the combined pill. When used perfectly, only about one woman in 200 will become pregnant each year (PEARL index 0.5). However, it works best about 4–6 hours after it is taken. If a couple prefer to have sex at night, after they have gone to bed, the best time to take the POP is late afternoon. This is easy to forget, and in the first year of use, about 5% of women find themselves pregnant because they have forgotten to take their pill, or taken it at an inappropriate time. Effectiveness is also more affected by vomiting and diarrhea, which prevents the absorption of the hormone (although the combined pill may also not work if women have been vomiting for more than 24 hours). An annoying side-effect in about 40% of women is that it makes periods irregular, leading to 'pregnancy scares'.

With both types of oral contraceptive, normal fertility almost always resumes once the medication is stopped.

'Depot' injections of progestagen

The commonest is 'depot Provera®' (medroxyprogesterone acetate). The injections have to be given by a nurse or doctor. Effectiveness lasts 6–10 weeks. During use, amenorrhea is common. However, there can be quite heavy bleeding as the effects wear off, or when the woman decides to stop using the method. However, the failure rate is only one per 300 women per year (PEARL index 0.3).

Post-coital contraception

These contain both estrogen and progestagen, at four times the dose of the ordinary combined pill. They need to be taken within 72 hours of intercourse. They can prevent up to 99% of pregnancies, depending on when they are taken. However, they cause vomiting in about 20% of women, and there is a particular concern about thrombosis because of the high dose of estrogen. Perhaps a better option for 'emergency' contraception is to insert a copper coil (IUCD). This can be done up to a week after intercourse and will prevent 999 out of 1000 pregnancies.

Sterilization

If a couple have decided that they never want to have children, or that their family is definitely complete, then sterilization is an option they should consider. It has the advantage of being permanent, with few if any long-term adverse effects. Both men and women can be sterilized, although it is more often the woman who chooses to be sterilized because she is the one who has the risk of being pregnant! If a woman with heart disease decides not to have children, her partner may wish to preserve his fertility in case he has another partner in the future. On the other hand, the risk of an operation is considerably less for a healthy partner than for someone with heart disease.

In current practice, most sterilizations are done with clips (or sometimes rings) applied to the fallopian tubes. This is done laparoscopically, but there is clearly a surgical and anesthetic risk that must be taken into account. The likelihood of pregnancy once the clips have been applied was traditionally quoted as one in 500, but recent studies suggest that the risk may be as high as 1%. Tubal ligation can be performed at cesarean section, but this procedure significantly increases the operative risk, and the chance of tubal recanalization is significantly higher than with interval elective laparoscopic sterilization.

If the man decides he should be sterilized, a vasectomy is performed. In the early years, reversal of sterilization is quite effective, but eventually in most men antisperm antibodies develop which impair the effectiveness of their sperm at fertilization. In such cases, intracytoplasmic sperm injection (ICSE) becomes necessary for conception.

In summary, when discussing contraception, couples should be assessed as individuals, taking into account the nature of the woman's cardiac lesion, her current medication, co-morbidities, any thrombotic tendency, and finally their personal preferences. One couple's perception of an acceptable risk may be unacceptable to another.

References and further reading

Burn J, Brennan P, Little J, *et al.* (1998) Recurrence risks in offspring of adults with major heart defects: results from first cohort of British collaborative study. *Lancet,* **351**, 311–316.

Carvalho JS (2001) Early prenatal diagnosis of major congenital heart defects. *Current Opinion in Obstetrics and Gynecology,* **13**, 155–159.

Hayman RG, Arulkumaran S & Steer PJ (2002) Uterine compression sutures: surgical management of postpartum hemorrhage. *Obstetrics and Gynecology,* **99**, 502–506.

Hyett J, Perdu M, Sharland G, Snijders R & Nicolaides KH (1999) Using fetal nuchal translucency to screen for major congenital cardiac defects at 10–14 weeks of gestation: population based cohort study. *British Medical Journal,* **318**, 81–85.

Lewis G & Drife JO (2004) *Why mothers die 2000–2002. Confidential enquiry into maternal and child health.* RCOG Press, London, UK. (http://www.cemach.org.uk/publications/WMD2000_2002/content.htm).

Lupton M, Oteng-Ntim E, Ayida G & Steer PJ (2002) Cardiac disease in pregnancy. *Current Opinion in Obstetrics and Gynecology,* **14**, 137–143.

Moons P, De Volder E, Budts W, *et al.* (2001) What do adult patients with congenital heart disease know about their disease, treatment, and prevention of complications? A call for structured patient education. *Heart,* **86**, 74–80.

Ramsey PS, Ramin KD & Ramin SM (2001) Cardiac disease in pregnancy. *American Journal of Perinatology,* **18**, 245–266.

Romano-Zelekha O, Hirsh R, Blieden L, Green M & Shohat T (2001) The risk for congenital heart defects in offspring of individuals with congenital heart defects. *Clinical Genetics,* **59**, 325–329.

Task Force on the Management of Cardiovascular Diseases During Pregnancy of the European Society of Cardiology (2003) Expert consensus document on management of cardiovascular diseases during pregnancy. *European Heart Journal,* **24**, 761–781.

CHAPTER 4

Infective Endocarditis Prophylaxis

Infective endocarditis (IE) denotes an infection of the endocardial surface of the heart or major vessels by microorganisms. Although the heart valves are most commonly affected, other sites can be involved in those with cardiac anomalies such as ventricular septal defect, patent ductus arteriosus and coarctation of the aorta.

Some features of IE have not changed over the past 30 years.
• The incidence remains at about 1.7–3.8 cases per 100,000 patient-years.
• Despite improvements in diagnosis and treatment, mortality remains high at approximately 20–25%. Death is primarily related to central nervous system embolic events and hemodynamic deterioration.
• The two essential risk factors for endocarditis are (1) structural abnormality of the heart or great arteries with significant pressure gradient or turbulent flow and (2) bacteremia.
• The oral cavity is still the primary source of bacteremia.
• Individuals with congenital heart anomalies are at increased risk for developing infective endocarditis and account for up to 20–35% of cases.

Other aspects have changed.
• While *Streptococcus viridans*, enterococci and *Staphylococcus aureus* still account for the majority of cases, an increasing number of more diverse organisms are involved (gram-negative, HACEK group, and fungal organisms).
• Median age has increased.
• Some treatment modalities have increased the number of patients at risk (immunosuppressive therapy with organ transplantation, cancer therapy, increased use of chronic in-dwelling central catheters, and surgery for congenital heart disease).

More children with congenital heart disease now survive into adulthood. The surgical procedures that have enabled them to live longer have two contrasting effects on the risk of IE. Certain operations eliminate or decrease the risk (repaired coarctation, ventricular septal defect and patent ductus arteriosus), while others increase the risk (prosthetic material and mechanical or bioprostheses). It is helpful to categorize the risk for IE of various unoperated and repaired congenital heart anomalies as (1) little or no risk, (2) moderate risk and (3) high risk. Endocarditis prophylaxis is not recommended in those at low level of risk, while it is recommended in those at moderate and high risk.

Little-or-no-risk category
• Atrial septal defect (ASD) (unoperated or repaired)

- Pulmonic stenosis, mild (unoperated or repaired)
- Repaired patent ductus arteriosus (PDA) and ventricular septal defect (VSD) without residual leak after 6 months
- Congenitally corrected transposition of the great arteries (TGA) (no associated lesions)
- Total or partial anomalous pulmonary venous return
- Coarctation of the aorta (unoperated) with small or absent gradient
- Ebstein anomaly (unoperated or repair of native valve)
- Cardiac pacemaker/implanted defibrillators

Moderate-risk category
- PDA and VSD with residual leak after repair
- Fontan repair
- Coarctation with more than mild obstruction
- Repaired defects including primum ASD with cleft mitral valve, complete atrioventricular septal defect, tetralogy of Fallot, TGA, truncus arteriosus
- Acquired valvular abnormalities (rheumatic)
- Mitral valve prolapse with valvular regurgitation/thickened leaflets
- Hypertrophic cardiomyopathy

High-risk category
- Prosthetic heart valves (mechanical, bioprosthesis and homograft)
- Previous IE
- Complex congenital heart disease with hypoxemia
- Surgically created systemic-to-pulmonary artery shunt or conduit
- VSD, unoperated
- Bicuspid aortic valve, aortic stenosis, sub-aortic stenosis

Endocarditis prophylaxis is recommended when patients in the moderate- and high-risk categories undergo procedures that place them at risk for significant or prolonged bacteremia. The major sources of bacteremia are the oral cavity, skin, genitourinary tract, reproductive tract, gastrointestinal tract, respiratory tract, and during surgery.

Dental procedures

Prophylaxis recommended	*Prophylaxis not recommended*
- Tooth extraction	- Local anesthetic injections, non-intraligamentary
- Restoration of decayed teeth	
- Peridontal procedures	- Post-procedure suture removal
- Dental implants	- Orthodontic appliance placement or adjustment
- Endodontic (root canal) procedures	
- Local anesthetic injection, intraligamentary	- Shedding of primary teeth
- Cleaning of teeth when bleeding is anticipated	- Taking of oral radiographs
	- Fluoride treatment

Genitourinary tract

Prophylaxis recommended
- Prostatic surgery
- Cystoscopy
- Urethral dilatation
- Urethral catheterization if infection present or traumatic
- Uterine dilatation and curettage, therapeutic abortion, sterilization procedure, insertion or removal of intrauterine device, especially if tissue infected

Prophylaxis not recommended
- Uncomplicated vaginal delivery
- Vaginal hysterectomy
- Cesarean section (debatable)
- Urethral catheterization, uterine dilatation and curettage, therapeutic abortion, sterilization procedure

Gastrointestinal tract

Prophylaxis recommended
- Dilatation of esophageal stricture
- Sclerotherapy for varices
- Biliary tract surgery or endoscopic procedure
- Surgery involving intestinal mucosa

Prophylaxis not recommended
- Endoscopic (upper or lower) with or without biopsy
- Transesophageal echocardiography

Respiratory tract

Prophylaxis recommended
- Tonsillectomy or adenoidectomy
- Surgical procedure involving the respiratory mucosa
- Bronchoscopy with rigid scope

Prophylaxis not recommended
- Endotracheal intubation
- Bronchoscopy with flexible scope with or without biopsy
- Tympanostomy tube insertion

Other procedures

Prophylaxis recommended
- 3–6-month period after reparative heart surgery for lesions that will qualify as low risk and not need prophylaxis
- Body piercing

Prophylaxis not recommended
- Cardiac catheterization including balloon angioplasty (debatable)
- Implanted cardiac pacemaker/defibrillator (debatable)
- Incision of surgically prepared skin
- Circumcision

Infective endocarditis prophylaxis

Prophylaxis involves education of individuals regarding both health mainte-nance and the need for antibiotic prophylaxis. All patients with congenital heart disease are encouraged to maintain good oral hygiene. This includes daily brushing and flossing of teeth as well as regular dental care. Dental prob-lems (decayed teeth, abscessed teeth and gum disease) should be promptly cared for. Good skin and nail care is important as this is a prime source of sta-phylococcus bacteremia. This includes avoiding biting of the skin around the nails and treatment of significant acne. Body piercing, especially involving the oral cavity or genitourinary system, puts individuals at risk for bacteremia.

The American Heart Association and the British Society for Antimicrobial Chemotherapy have published guidelines for antibiotic prophylaxis based on the risk categories, type of procedure and likely organisms that will get into the bloodstream. While it is acknowledged that no adequate controlled trials are available that confirm the efficacy of antibiotic prophylaxis against endo-carditis, it seems prudent in individuals who have cardiac abnormalities that increase their risk.

The recommended antibiotics for endocarditis prophylaxis are listed in the table below. The American Heart Association has a pocket-size card outlining its recommendations that can be given to patients.

Prophylactic regimens

Dental, oral, respiratory tract, or esophageal procedures

Situation	Agent	Dosage
Standard	Amoxicillin	Adult: 2.0 g orally 1 hour before procedure
Unable to take oral medications	Ampicillin	Adult: 2.0 g IM or IV within 30 minutes before procedure
Allergic to penicillin	Clindamycin	Adult: 600 mg orally 1 hour before procedure
	Cefalexin or cefadroxil	Adult: 2.0 g orally 1 hour before procedure
	Azithromycin or clarithromycin	Adult: 500 mg orally 1 hour before procedure
Unable to take oral medications and allergic to penicillin	Clindamycin	Adult: 600 mg IV within 30 minutes before procedure
	Cefazolin	Adult: 1.0 g IM or IV within 30 minutes before procedure

Genitourinary and gastrointestinal tract procedures

Situation	Agent	Dosage
High-risk patients	Ampicillin plus gentamicin	Adults: ampicillin 2.0 g IM or IV plus gentamicin 1.5 mg/kg (not to exceed 120 mg) within 30 minutes of starting the procedure. In addition, ampicillin 1.0 g IM or IV or amoxicillin 1.0 g orally 6 hours later
High-risk patients allergic to ampicillin or amoxicillin	Vancomycin plus gentamicin	Adults: vancomycin 1.0 g IV over 1–2 hours plus gentamicin 1.5 mg/ kg IV or IM (not to exceed 120 mg) with administration of medication completed within 30 minutes of starting procedure
Moderate-risk patients	Amoxicillin or ampicillin	Adults: amoxicillin 2.0 g orally 1 hour before procedure or ampicillin 2.0 g IM or IV within 30 minutes of starting the procedure
Moderate-risk patients allergic to ampicillin or amoxicillin	Vancomycin	Adults: vancomycin 1.0 g IV over 1–2 hours; complete infusion within 30 minutes of starting procedure

Key clinical points

• Infective endocarditis still has significant morbidity and mortality despite current diagnostic and therapeutic options.
• Endocarditis prevention focuses on health maintenance and antibiotics given prior to procedures that cause significant bacteremia in individuals at risk for developing IE.
• Individuals with congenital heart disease should be educated on issues related to care of teeth and skin to decrease the risk of IE.
• Those in moderate- and high-risk categories should be informed for what procedures antibiotic prophylaxis is advised and provided with a card outlining current antibiotic recommendations.

Further reading

Bayer AS, Bolger AF, Taubert KA, *et al.* (1988) Diagnosis and management of infective endocarditis and its complications. *Circulation*, **98**, 2936–2948.

Dajani AS, Taubert KA, Wilson, *et al.* (1997) Prevention of bacterial endocarditis. Recommendations by the American Heart Association. *Circulation*, **96**, 358–366 and *Journal of the American Medical Association*, **277**, 1794–1801.

Gersony WM, Hayes CJ, Driscoll DJ, *et al.* (1993) Bacterial endocarditis in patients with aortic stenosis, pulmonary stenosis, or ventricular septal defect. *Circulation*, **87** (Suppl I), I-121–I-126.

Morris CD, Reller MD & Menashe VD (1998) Thirty-year incidence of infective endocarditis after surgery for congenital heart disease. *Journal of the American Medical Association*, **279**, 599–603.

Mylonakis E & Calderwood S (2001) Infective endocarditis in adults. *New England Journal of Medicine*, **345**, 1318–1330.

Working Party of the British Society for Antimicrobial Chemotherapy (1998) Antibiotic treatment of streptococcal, enterococcal, and staphylococcal endocarditis. *Heart*, **79**, 207–210.

CHAPTER 5

Anticoagulation

In adults with congenital heart disease, anticoagulation and antiplatelet therapy may be necessary to prevent thrombosis or embolism related to:

- mechanical or bioprosthetic valves;
- supraventricular arrhythmia;
- cardioversion;
- issues specific to congenital heart disease:
  - Blalock-Taussig shunt,
  - Fontan circulation,
  - cyanosis,
  - Eisenmenger syndrome,
  - conduits, stents and closure devices.

In addition, those on chronic anticoagulation therapy require adjustment during:

- surgery;
- pregnancy.

Prosthetic and native valve disease

Mechanical valves

All patients with a mechanical valve should receive warfarin therapy if possible. The following table outlines recommendations.

Type of valve	Recommendation
Aortic valve	Warfarin (INR 2.0–3.0)
Aortic valve + AF	Warfarin (INR 2.5–3.5) or INR 2.0–3.0 plus low-dose aspirin
Mitral valve +/- AF	Warfarin (INR 2.5–3.5)
Caged ball type prosthesis	Warfarin (INR 2.5–3.5) plus low-dose aspirin

If an embolus occurs despite adequate INR, two options are to add low-dose aspirin or increase the INR to the next higher therapeutic range. For individuals unable to take aspirin, alternatives are dipyridamole or clopidogrel.

Bioprosthetic valve

Recommended therapy for bioprosthetic valves is outlined below.

Type of valve	Recommendation
Mitral valve	Warfarin (INR 2.0–3.0) for 3 months, then low-dose aspirin
Aortic valve	Low-dose aspirin
Aortic or mitral valve with AF	Warfarin (INR 2.0–3.0)
Pulmonary or tricuspid valve	Low-dose aspirin for at least 3 months

Supraventricular arrhythmias

If intermittent or chronic atrial flutter or fibrillation occurs, the necessity for anticoagulation therapy needs to be considered. Certain factors predict a high risk for embolic events in association with atrial flutter or fibrillation. These include a previous stroke/TIA or other systemic emboli, hypertension, poor systemic ventricular function and age.

Recommendations for anticoagulation therapy for intermittent or chronic atrial fibrillation suggest warfarin (INR 2–3) for those with risk factors and high-dose aspirin for those at lesser risk.

Electrical cardioversion

When electrical cardioversion for atrial flutter/fibrillation is indicated, recommendations are as follows:
• Minimum of warfarin (INR 2–3) for 3 weeks before and 4 weeks after cardioversion.
• For urgent cardioversion, IV heparin is given as soon as possible, then a transesophageal echocardiogram. Cardioversion can be performed if no thrombus is seen. Warfarin is continued for at least 4 weeks after cardioversion.
• For atrial flutter/fibrillation of less than 48 hours duration, IV heparin is given during the peri-cardioversion period and warfarin for at least 4 weeks afterwards. The need for long-term warfarin or aspirin needs to be addressed in all patients undergoing a cardioversion.

Issues specific for congenital heart disease

Blalock-Taussig shunt

Although the use of palliative systemic-to-pulmonary shunts has decreased, the modified Blalock-Taussig shunt with a Gore-Tex® tube graft continues to be performed. Some use heparin during the perioperative period followed by aspirin to reduce the risk of acute shunt thrombosis.

Fontan circulation

After Fontan surgery, individuals have increased risk of venous thrombosis and emboli to either the lungs or the systemic circulation (incidence of 3–19%). This may occur at any time following surgery, but no predisposing factors have been clearly identified. The efficacy of anticoagulation in reducing the thrombotic risk has not been proven in clinical trials. Consequently, different approaches are taken. Some advocate warfarin for the first few months after surgery followed by long-term aspirin. Others just use long-term aspirin. Some centers taking care of adults recommend that all who have had a Fontan procedure take warfarin, especially old-style Fontans.

Another indication for anticoagulant therapy in the Fontan patient is protein-losing enteropathy (PLE). Low-dose, subcutaneous heparin (5,000 units/ day) can improve or reverse the abnormalities associated with PLE. The benefit is not due to the anticoagulant effects of the heparin, but possibly to stabilization of the capillary endothelium.

Cyanotic patients

These patients have both a bleeding and a thrombotic diathesis. The bleeding diathesis is due to:

- decreased vitamin K-dependent clotting factors;
- thrombocytopenia;
- platelet dysfunction;
- von Willebrand-like abnormality;
- increased fibrinolytic activity.

These coagulation abnormalities are evident by prolongation of activated partial thromboplastin time (APTT), INR and bleeding time. Mucosal bleeding and easy bruising are the most frequent problems. Bleeding can be dramatic and life-threatening with hemoptysis and intrapulmonary hemorrhage. Anticoagulation and antiplatelet agents should be avoided and bleeding treated, if necessary, by correcting the specific abnormality causing the problem. Those with cyanosis are also at risk for venous thrombosis, pulmonary arterial thrombosis and systemic emboli. Cyanotic patients frequently develop atrial fibrillation, another predisposing factor for embolism. Since anticoagulation therapy is high risk, indications for its use should be strong and well documented.

Achieving the desired INR can be difficult. The cyanotic individual may be very sensitive to warfarin. Measuring the INR when the hematocrit is elevated is problematic. Blood is drawn into a tube with a fixed volume of anticoagulant. The amount of anticoagulant in the tube, normally suitable for a hematocrit in the normal range, is excessive for the volume of plasma when the hematocrit is elevated. This excessive dilution of the plasma gives a falsely elevated value.

Eisenmenger syndrome

In primary pulmonary hypertension, microvascular and macrovascular thrombosis increase morbidity and mortality. Anticoagulation therapy effectively reduces these risks. Since a similar pulmonary pathology is present in Eisenmenger syndrome, some advocate routine warfarin anticoagulation for these patients. Others feel that anticoagulation should be used only in the presence of venous thrombosis, embolic events, or atrial flutter/fibrillation.

No clinical trials are available to support routine anticoagulation use in Eisenmenger syndrome.

Conduits, stents, and closure devices

Stents are used to manage branch stenosis of the branch pulmonary arteries, pulmonary vein stenosis, coarctation of the aorta, and stenoses related to surgery. Heparin is given at the time of insertion followed by aspirin for a period of months (usually 3–6 months).

The most effective, low-risk therapy to prevent thrombus on these closure devices has not been adequately established. Various approaches are currently used, but are likely to evolve as experience increases. The majority of units use a combination of peri-procedural heparin followed by aspirin and/or clopidogrel.

Management of anticoagulation in the perioperative period

Patients receiving chronic anticoagulation therapy need to have their anticoagulation interrupted when undergoing a surgical procedure. Most surgeries can be done safely with an INR <1.5. While there is no consensus on the optimal management, the following guidelines are suggested.

In patients at low risk for thrombus taking warfarin with an INR in the therapeutic range the protocol is as follows:

- Withhold 4 scheduled doses of warfarin.
- Check INR the day prior to surgery.
- If >1.5, a small dose of oral or subcutaneous vitamin K can be given.
- Warfarin can be started the day after surgery if bleeding risk is low or as soon as safely possible. The INR usually returns to the therapeutic range by the third day.

With this protocol, the patient is sub-therapeutic for 2 days prior to surgery and at least 2 days after surgery. During the days after surgery when the INR is less than 2.0, subcutaneous heparin can be given.

Those at high risk for thrombus are usually fully anticoagulated with intravenous heparin perioperatively. The heparin can be stopped 6 hours prior to surgery and restarted without a bolus 12 hours after surgery if bleeding is not a concern.

Management of anticoagulation during pregnancy

Anticoagulation may be necessary during pregnancy for therapy of venous thromboembolism or to prevent thrombus on a mechanical heart valve. Risks to both the mother and fetus need to be considered. The maternal risks are bleeding, osteoporosis and thrombocytopenia. The fetal complications are spontaneous abortion, stillbirth, premature delivery, teratogenesis and bleeding. Some risks are agent-specific.

Unfractionated heparin (UFH), low molecular-weight heparin (LMWH) and warfarin are three anticoagulants used during pregnancy. The use of LMWH rather than UFH is attractive due to its superior bioavailability, ease of use and reduced risk of osteoporosis. Problems include the uncertainty of dosage and how best to monitor therapy. Thrombotic events and deaths have been reported with use of LMWH during pregnancy. Hopefully, additional data will be available soon that establish whether LMWH is a safe and effective anticoagulant to use during pregnancy.

Maternal risks
- Warfarin
  - Changing dose requirements during the pregnancy.
  - Half-life is days.
- Heparin
  - Variable response to standard dose.
  - Short half-life (60 minutes).
  - APTT results can be variable.
  - Osteoporosis and risk of fractures. LMWH has a much lower risk of osteoporosis than heparin.
  - Heparin tends to decrease platelet count to some degree, although the risk of heparin-induced thrombocytopenia is low at 3%. This is defined as a platelet count below 100,000 or a fall to <50% of baseline. Low normal or low platelets counts are present in many patients with congenital heart disease.
  - Risk of valve thrombosis.

Fetal risks
- Warfarin
  - Crosses the placenta, increasing the risk of bleeding (may be fatal) and teratogenesis (risk = 6.4%).
  - Embryopathy (nasal hypoplasia, microcephaly and stippled epiphyses) is highest in the first trimester, especially between 6 and 12 weeks.
  - Embryopathy risk may be minimal with low doses (less than 5 mg/day).
  - No anticoagulant effect has been found in infants being breastfed by mothers taking warfarin.
- Heparin
  - Since neither UFH nor LMWH cross the placenta, bleeding or teratogenesis in the fetus are not an issue. Bleeding at the uteroplacental junction is possible.
  - Infants are not affected by anticoagulation used by a nursing mother. UFH and LMWH are not secreted into breast milk.

Recommendations
Women of childbearing age on long-term warfarin therapy need to be counseled about the risks of anticoagulation during pregnancy. These risks are not inconsequential and include maternal mortality of 2.9%, major bleeding

(2.9%) and thrombus/embolus (3.9%). If a pregnancy is planned, one of two approaches to anticoagulation can be selected.

• Perform frequent pregnancy tests and switch to UFH when pregnancy is detected. This approach assumes that warfarin is safe during the first 4–6 weeks of pregnancy.

• An alternative approach is to switch to UFH before pregnancy (during the time the woman is trying to become pregnant). The disadvantage of this approach is the more prolonged use of UFH and increased risk for an osteoporotic fracture.

Once pregnancy is confirmed (usually by 6 weeks) in a woman receiving long-term warfarin, three options are available.

• UFH from the time pregnancy is identified through 12 weeks, returning to warfarin use, and switching back to heparin close to term. This approach provides the lowest risk of valve thrombosis or systemic emboli. The recommended INR range during pregnancy is 2.5–3.5.

• Continue warfarin even after the pregnancy is confirmed and switch to heparin close to term. This approach may be the best option if the warfarin dosage during pregnancy will be ≤5 mg/day. These low doses pose little or no risk for embryopathy, although the risk of fetal bleeding is still present.

• Heparin throughout pregnancy. This approach avoids the risk of warfarin embroypathy, but is the least effective at preventing thrombus or emboli.

Aspirin

• Potential risks include bleeding in the woman or fetus and birth defects (overall very small).

• Low-dose aspirin during the second and third trimester is safe.

• The safety of higher doses is uncertain.

• No data are available regarding the risk/benefit of addition of low-dose aspirin to warfarin or heparin during pregnancy.

Key clinical points

• Anticoagulation therapy may be indicated for:
  – mechanical or bioprosthetic valves;
  – rheumatic mitral valve disease;
  – supraventricular arrhythmia;
  – cardioversion.
• Anticoagulation may be needed in adults with congenital heart disease under the following circumstances:
  – Blalock-Taussig shunt, Fontan circulation;
  – cyanosis, Eisenmenger syndrome;
  – conduits, stents, and closure devices.
• Recommendations are outlined for anticoagulation management during non-cardiac surgery in individuals who require long-term anticoagulation therapy.

- Management of anticoagulation during pregnancy is a balance of risk/benefit to the mother and fetus.
- Knowledge of the interaction of other medications with warfarin, heparin and aspirin is essential to their safe and effective use.

Further reading

Albers GW, Dalen JE, Laupacis A, Manning WJ, Petersen P & Singer DE (2001) Antithrombotic therapy in atrial fibrillation. *Chest*, **119**, 194S–206S.

Ginsberg JS, Greer I & Hirsh J (2001) Use of antithrombotic agents during pregnancy. *Chest*, **119**, 112S–131S.

Kearon C & Hirsh J (1977) Management of anticoagulation before and after elective surgery. *New England Journal of Medicine*, **336**, 1506–1511.

Monagle P, Michelson AD, Bovill E & Andrew M (2001) Antithrombotic therapy in children. *Chest*, **119**, 344S–370S.

Reller MD (2001) Congenital heart disease: current indications for antithrombotic therapy in pediatric patients. *Current Cardiology Reports*, **3**, 90–95.

Stein PD, Alpert JS, Bussey HI, Dalen JE & Turpie AGG (2001) Antithrombotic therapy in patients with mechanical and biological prosthetic heart valves. *Chest*, **119**, 220S–227S.

Vitale N, De Feo M, De Santo LS, Pollice A, Tedesco N & Cotrufo M (1999) Dose-dependent fetal complications of warfarin in pregnant women with mechanical heart valves. *Journal of the American College of Cardiology*, **33**, 1637–1641.

Wells PS, Holbrook AM, Crowther NR, *et al.* (1994) Interaction of warfarin with drugs and food: a critical review of the literature. *Annals of Internal Medicine*, **121**, 676–683.

CHAPTER 6

Lifestyle Issues

Exercise

Exercise capacity has been shown to be greatly diminished in patients with congenital heart disease, whether 'unrepaired' or 'repaired'. Maximum oxygen uptake is about half the predicted normal level for age and sex and diminishes with age. Factors responsible for a diminished exercise capacity are thought to include diminished vital capacity, chronotopic incompetence, decreased ventricular function, as well as abnormal sympathetic and parasympathetic response to exercise.

Exercise rehabilitation programs in stable patients with congenital heart disease show some benefits, with improvements of maximum oxygen consumption.

Recommendations for exercise prescription in adult patients with congenital heart disease are detailed in a consensus report from 1994 and summarized below.

No restriction in physical activity	Restricted physical activity to class IA type activities (low static and low dynamic impact)	Contraindication to physical activity
Patients with left-to-right shunting lesions with normal pulmonary pressure and no cardiomegaly	Patients with left-to-right shunting lesions and some degree of pulmonary hypertension or cardiomegaly	Patients with severe pulmonary hypertension

Patients with severe cardiomegaly |
| Patients with mild right-sided or left-sided obstructive lesions (mild pulmonary stenosis (PS), mild aortic stenosis (AS) and mild coarctation of the aorta) | Patients with moderate to severe obstructive lesions

Patients with clinically stable repaired tetralogy of fallot, Mustard, arterial switch, Ebstein and the Fontan procedure | Patients with life-threatening arrhythmias

Patients with class IV symptoms |

Although the recommendations for the permitted level of activity presented in the 1994 American College of Cardiology document are helpful, they are intended to be used as a guideline only, with the understanding that a physician with knowledge of a particular patient's lesion severity and physiologic response to exercise may choose to modify these recommendations accordingly, on a case-by-case basis.

Appropriate advice regarding exercise prescription for these patients is important but often neglected at the time of routine clinical visits. Without proper guidance, low-risk patients will limit their physical activities unduly, while high-risk patients may engage in improper high-risk physical activities. Education of patients regarding the type of exercise they can safely perform is paramount.

Work and insurance

Work

Vocational choices for the adolescent with congenital heart disease (CHD) are important issues that need to be addressed in a timely fashion. There are two aspects that need to be discussed.

• The patient's physical ability to match the demands of a given occupation, without compromising cardiovascular wellbeing. This largely, but not solely, depends on the type of CHD defect, the effects of previous intervention(s) and anticipated long-term outcomes.

• The question as to whether to choose a career that would enhance the chances for recruitment by larger employers who often provide health, disability and/or life insurance through group policies. This is of particular relevance for patients with moderate to severe forms of CHD, normally deemed uninsurable or having to pay very high premiums (see also Insurability below).

In general, the following applies.

• Patients with small or repaired septal defects or PDAs and those with mild pulmonary stenosis do not require any occupational restrictions.

• Patients with moderate CHD or CHD which is progressive in nature may require tailoring of their jobs, generally towards white-collar occupations.

• Patients with major CHD such as severe left-sided obstructive lesions, aortic dilatation, advanced myocardial dysfunction, single ventricle physiology and more than mild pulmonary vascular disease clearly need to be restricted from high-risk occupations. These patients are unsuitable for physically demanding jobs or employment on which the lives of others are directly dependent (for example, pilots or heavy equipment operators).

Informed counseling of patients (during early adolescence) and their families on this sensitive issue enables appropriate career planning and overcomes unrealistic expectations, and occasionally allows patients with relatively minor defects to consider wider career options. Clearly, the right balance needs to be achieved between discussing the realities of the patient's condition and applying too much pressure on young individuals. It is our personal impression that most patients and families welcome such an initiative and are relieved when this important matter is brought up for discussion.

Insurability

A number of large-scale, long-term studies are available for prognostication of outcomes in many congenital heart lesions. This has facilitated estimation of mortality risks compared to healthy control populations, which in turn is the basis of life insurance policies. Among the most important of these studies is a report from the pediatric cardiac surgical database of 6,461 children operated in Finland between the years 1953 and 1989. After exclusion of perioperative mortality, the late mortality rate over 45 years among congenital heart patients as a group was 16%, compared to 7% for an age, time and sex-matched population. Mortality rates for specific lesions with up to five decades of follow-up after surgery were calculated and ranged between 5% for atrial septal defects to 85% for patients with single ventricle physiology.

In general terms, prognosis can be grouped as follows.

• Lesions with a good outcome (normal or near normal prognosis): atrial septal defect (ASD), ventricular septal defect (VSD), patent ductus arteriosus (PDA), and pulmonary stenosis.

• Lesions with an intermediate outcome (residual hemodynamic abnormalities and therefore a more guarded prognosis): aortic stenosis, tetralogy of Fallot and transposition after the Mustard or Senning procedure.

• Lesions with an uncertain or poor outcome (complex uncorrected anatomy, large variability between individuals with the same lesion, and/or limited data to guide prognosis); transposition of great arteries after the arterial switch procedure, congenitally corrected transposition, Ebstein's anomaly and single ventricle physiology.

For purposes of life insurance, companies consider the expected mortality of a given patient group compared to the observed mortality in a reference population (usually a cohort of insured individuals of the same age) in order to derive a mortality ratio. For example, patients whose mortality rate is the same as a reference population have a mortality ratio of 100%, while patients with a mortality rate of 5% over 10 years, compared to a reference population rate of 1% over 10 years, have a mortality ratio of 500%. For each 100% increase in mortality ratio, the premium paid for insurance is increased by approximately 90%. Patients with a predicted mortality ratio >500% are rarely considered insurable.

Prognosis varies within individual lesions. For example, patients with tetralogy of Fallot as a whole have a reduced survival rate compared to healthy controls. However, patients repaired early, not requiring a transannular patch, without significant pulmonary stenosis or regurgitation and a short QRS on their EKG have a long-term prognosis which is not different from normal. A good to excellent prognosis can also be expected in a number of lesions when present in mild form, not requiring surgery or other intervention. In general, the presence of biventricular circulation and a systemic left ventricle, repair at early age, good functional capacity and the absence of major or progressive hemodynamic lesions are positive prognostic markers and need to be emphasized when physicians are asked to produce a supportive letter for insurance purposes.

Guidelines for patients and physicians
• Declined patients or those offered insurance at high premiums should shop around, as not all companies rate risk the same.

• The local adult CHD patient association may be able to provide advice about insurers with a track record of providing coverage for this growing patient population.

• One important avenue for obtaining health, disability and/or life insurance is through group insurance policies available through employers or professional associations. Group policies do not require an individual evaluation, as they are based on the assumption that the majority of an unselected employee group or association will be healthy. Hence, even adult patients with complex CHD may obtain insurance via this route, without the need for individual assessment.

• Another product that may be available in certain places is the non-renewable term policy, which provides short-term coverage ending after a fixed period of time (usually 10 years). These may be useful to some patients until the natural history of their congenital lesion is better understood.

• Finally, other factors, especially age and smoking status, affect insurability. Since mortality in the general population predictably increases with age, whereas the mortality associated with a congenital heart defect may remain the same, mortality ratios of congenital heart patients inevitably decrease with age. Hence, those who were uninsurable at age 30 may be able to obtain coverage after age 50. Avoidance of smoking and adoption of good health practices will lower a patient's overall risk, and further increase their chances of insurability. Attention to reducing coronary risk factors to a minimum is more likely to allow a favorable insurance decision.

Key points

• Vocational choice for the adolescent with CHD depends on the type of defect, previous intervention(s) and long-term outcomes.

• Like the general population, adult patients with CHD desire the financial security that comes with insurance.

• Patients with repaired ASD, PDA, PS and VSD with low mortality ratios should be able to obtain insurance without problem.

• Patients with intermediate prognosis lesions represent a higher-risk group to insurers, but may achieve insurance on the basis of individual consideration, especially in the absence of negative prognostic features.

• Patients with uncertain or poor prognosis lesions, such as those with complex CHD, will for the most part be considered uninsurable on an individual basis. However, alternative routes via group policies may exist.

• With newer surgical and catheter techniques, advancing medical therapy and improved risk stratification, overall prognosis and hence insurability will continue to improve for adults with CHD.

Table 6.1 summarizes currently published mortality data for common defects from a variety of sources. In addition, where permitted by available data, the best-case scenario mortality rates are shown for low-risk patients within each anatomical subgroup. Also shown for each lesion are mortality ratios calculated from the published mortality rates in patients compared to their reference popu-

Table 6.1 Mortality rates for operated congenital heart lesions compared to a reference population. (Where permitted by available data, mortality in low-risk subgroups within each lesion are shown)

Lesion	Reference #	Duration of follow-up (years)	Late mortality all patients* (%)	Late mortality low-risk subgroup (%)	Mortality in reference population (%)	Mortality ratio all patients** (%)	Mortality ratio low-risk subgroup** (%)	Mortality ratio in insurance underwriting manuals§ (%)
Patent ductus arteriosus	5	45	12†	N/A	6	200	N/A	100
Pulmonary stenosis	10	25	10	6‡	6‡	167	100	100 up
Ventricular septal defect	7	27	20	5	3	667	167	100–200
Coarctation of the aorta	8	20	16†	9†	5‡	320	180	100–300
Aortic stenosis	11	25	15†	8†	4	375	200	225–400 up
Tetralogy of Fallot	12	32	14	7	4	350	175	200–400
Senning/Mustard	15	20	24	N/A	5††	480	N/A	Declined
Single ventricle	4	34	85†	N/A	3‡	>2800	N/A	Declined

* Excludes surgical mortality unless otherwise indicated.

** Calculated as mortality rate in patients/mortality rate in reference population × 100.

§ Range of mortality ratios published by three insurance companies in underwriting manuals; calculated as mortality rate in patients/mortality rate in reference population of insured individuals × 100 [4].

† Includes surgical mortality.

‡ Mortality rate estimated from Kaplan Meier curve.

†† No reference population rate given; mortality rate estimated from other studies.

For details refer to source.

N/A Not available from published data.

Reproduced with permission from Vonder-Muhll I *et al.* (2003) *European Heart Journal,* **25**, 1595–1600.

lation. For comparison purposes, the last column shows the range of mortality ratios quoted in three insurance underwriting manuals.

Travel

Physicians are frequently asked by patients with chronic heart disease whether they can safely travel. Questions usually relate to commercial aircraft travel or visiting locations at higher elevations. Concerns, especially during commercial aircraft travel, include:
- hypoxemia, especially in cyanotic patients;
- venous thromboembolism;
- physical and emotional stress of travel;
- risk of cardiac events and death;
- exposure to other illnesses:
    - gastroenteritis,
    - upper respiratory tract infections,
    - other infectious diseases.

Hypoxemia
- Commercial aircraft cabins are pressurized to 6000–8000 feet (1829–2438 meters).
- Healthy people have little difficulty in adapting to the decrease in ambient oxygen and compensate by increasing ventilation. This moderates the average fall in arterial oxygen saturation of about 8 percentage points.
- Patients with cyanotic congenital heart disease also have a similar 8 percentage points decrease from their baseline oxygen saturation, but tolerate this well without supplemental oxygen. They maintain adequate tissue oxygen delivery due to the chronic rightward shift in their oxyhemoglobin dissociation curve and to secondary erythrocytosis. Inflight inhaled oxygen is rarely indicated.

Venous thrombosis
- Venous thrombosis and embolism are a risk with any form of prolonged travel. The mechanism is stasis in the venous circulation of the lower limbs.
- The incidence is uncertain, but the overall risk is small.
- Venous thrombosis is rarely observed after flights of <5 hours. The incidence increases with flights ≥12 hours.
- Symptoms of thromboembolism may develop during or immediately after the flight, but more commonly occur 1 to 3 days after travel.
- Risk factors for venous thrombosis include age >50, previous venous thrombosis, thrombophilic abnormality, CHF, obesity, prolonged immobility, dehydration, estrogen therapy and pregnancy.
- General preventive measures are as follows.
    - If possible, delay travel if the risk factor for venous thrombosis will decrease over a short time period (e.g. recovery from surgery).
    - Regularly change position and walk when possible.

 – Perform leg exercises during prolonged sitting (flexion, extension, and rotation of ankles).
 – Maintain hydration. It is not necessary to abstain from alcohol, but it does promote diuresis and inactivity.
 – It is not necessary to stop BCP or HRT unless the risk of venous thrombosis is increased.
• Additional preventive measures may be considered for individuals judged at increased risk for venous thrombosis.
 – Below-knee elastic stockings properly fitted.
 – Aspirin; while the value of aspirin against venous thrombosis is uncertain, some data do suggest a benefit in preventing venous thrombosis.
 – Heparin is considered in the infrequent individual at high risk for thrombus (e.g. previous venous thrombosis). A single subcutaneous injection of LMWH a few hours before the flight should be sufficient in almost all cases.

Physical and emotional stress of travel
In people with limited exercise capacity, the following options may help reduce the physical and emotional stress of traveling.
• The actual flight is rarely physically stressful, but can be fatiguing. It may be helpful to schedule a rest day between connections of a very long trip.
• Ensure transportation in the airport, especially between connecting flights.
• Arrange for porters to transport luggage.
• A companion traveler may be desirable to provide reassurance and assistance.

Serious events
Serious events are rare, but little data are available about the actual number of events.
• Death during a flight is very rare.
• Acute myocardial infarction in flight is infrequent and does not appear to relate to hypoxemia.
• Acute pulmonary emboli may cause acute symptoms and accounted for 18% of deaths that occurred either inflight or shortly after arrival to a single major airport.
• Individuals with a history of arrhythmias may have an event precipitated by the stress of travel.

Specific situations
Development of high-altitude pulmonary edema during air travel is a rare event. An association between high-altitude pulmonary edema (HAPE) in children with Down syndrome has been reported during rapid ascent to moderate elevation (1738–3252 meters). It is uncertain whether this risk translates to air travel for these individuals, as the cabin pressure would be in this same range.

Driving

In contrast to the low risk of travel, driving a motorized vehicle is an inherently dangerous activity with associated significant mortality and morbidity. Societies have accepted these risks in order to have the freedom and lifestyle alternatives that motor vehicles provide. Societies have also determined that driving privileges should be restricted in those people who are likely to place themselves and others at unacceptable risk. The level of risk chosen varies between countries and even between states in the USA. A distinction is also made between types of drivers. Those who drive large trucks, large passenger-carrying vehicles (buses, subways or trains) and smaller passenger-carrying vehicles such as a taxi must conform to stricter standards compared with those who drive a small personal vehicle.

Physicians are frequently consulted to judge whether a specific medical illness should lead to driving restrictions. The medical communities in Canada, the USA and Europe have published guidelines for patients with various cardiovascular abnormalities (see Further reading). The overriding concern is that a medical problem may increase the individual's risk to drive due to a sudden loss of consciousness or significant alteration of mental awareness. Some general concepts are important to consider.

• Driver errors, excessive speed for the conditions, and excessive alcohol intake are by far the most important factors that lead to death and injury due to driving.

• The corollary to this is that the medical condition of the driver is an uncommon factor in accidents involving injury or death. Sudden driver incapacity due to a medical illness occurs in approximately 1 per 1,000 accidents resulting in injury or death.

• In the people who became incapacitated while driving due to a medical illness, most continued to drive despite a recent similar incapacitating event.

In most societies, any episode of loss of consciousness or significant alteration of mental status disqualifies an individual from driving. After such an episode, the person should not drive until he or she has undergone an appropriate medical evaluation. The more common etiologies identified as likely causes are:

• neurocardiogenic or vasovagal syncope;
• seizures;
• tachyarrhythmias (supraventricular and ventricular);
• bradyarrhythmias.

Less common etiologies include hypoglycemia, acute myocardial infarction or prolonged severe anginal episode, stroke and carotid sinus syndrome. Despite a thorough evaluation, no etiology will be established in up to 20% of cases.

Various therapies or procedures designed to prevent recurrent syncope are available. The issue for the physician is to determine when it is safe for the patient to resume driving after therapy has been initiated to prevent recurrent loss of consciousness. Two general methods are used for determining effectiveness of therapy. First, a test can be done to establish efficacy. For arrhythmias, this may include electrophysiologic testing or prolonged EKG event monitoring. The second, and more commonly applied method, assumes a reasonable degree of efficacy after the patient is observed for a specific period of time without recurrence of the event.

The following table provides recommendations for small vehicle driving after initiation of therapy or procedures designed to prevent recurrent syncopal episodes. The recommendations cover issues most likely to be seen in the adult with CHD. These are guidelines based on sparse data and not standards of practice. The recommendations will change as better information becomes available.

Cause of impaired consciousness	Recommendation for driving
Seizure	After 6 months if no recurrence
Ventricular tachycardia (VT)/ fibrillation (VF)	After 6 months if either no recurrence or no impairment of consciousness with arrhythmia
Automatic implantable cardiac defibrillator (AICD) placement for VT/VF	After 6 months if no impairment of consciousness with arrhythmias or at time of AICD discharge; after 1 week if AICD was placed prophylactically in a high-risk patient without VT/VF event
Supraventricular tachycardia	After 1 month if either no recurrence or no impairment of consciousness with arrhythmia
Bradycardia	1 week after either pacemaker insertion or removal of cause of bradycardia (e.g. medications)
Neurally mediated syncope with mild symptoms	No restrictions
Neurally mediated syncope with severe symptoms	After 3 months if either no symptoms or only mild symptoms
Cause not established	After 3 months if no recurrence of loss or impairment of consciousness

Key clinical points

Travel

- Travel is generally very safe for people with CHD.
- The reduced oxygen content in the cabins of commercial aircraft is well tolerated even by those with cyanotic CHD. Inflight oxygen is rarely required for chronically hypoxemic people.
- Venous thrombosis is a risk during prolonged flights (>12 hours) and in people with known risk factors.

• General measures to prevent venous thrombosis include frequently changing position, leg exercises if prolonged sitting is required, and maintaining adequate hydration.
• Additional preventive measure such as below-knee elastic stockings, aspirin, or rarely, LMWH, are considered in people identified at high risk for venous thrombosis.

Driving

• Driving a motor vehicle is an inherently dangerous activity that societies have accepted in order to have the freedom and lifestyle alternatives this provides.
• Most deaths and injuries related to driving are due to driver error, excessive speed and excessive alcohol intake.
• A medical condition that causes loss of consciousness of the driver is an uncommon cause of an accident (estimated at 1 in 1,000 accidents).
• Any loss of consciousness or significant alteration of mental status should disqualify an individual from driving and prompt a thorough medical evaluation to seek the etiology.
• Most common causes of loss of consciousness are neurocardiogenic or vasovagal syncope, seizures, supraventricular and ventricular tachycardias, and bradyarrhythmias. No etiology for the event can be identified in up to 20% of cases.
• Most people can resume driving if episodes of loss of consciousness or altered mental status do not recur after an appropriate period of observation.

Further reading

Exercise

Fredriksen PM, Veldtman G, Hechter S, *et al.* (2001) Aerobic capacity in adults with various congenital heart diseases. *American Journal of Cardiology*, **87**, 310–314.

Graham TP, Bricker JT, James FW, *et al.* (1994) Task Force 1: Congenital Heart Disease I. *Journal of the American College of Cardiology*, **24**, 845–899.

Swan L & Hillis WS (2000) Exercise prescription in adults with congenital heart disease: a long way to go. *Heart*, **83**, 685–687.

Therrien J, Fredriksen PM, Walder M, *et al.* (2003) A pilot study of exercise training in adult patients with repaired tetralogy of Fallot. *Canadian Journal of Cardiology*, **19**, 685–689.

Work and insurance

Cumming GR (2001) Insurance issues in adults with congenital heart disease. In *Diagnosis and Management of Adult Congenital Heart Disease* (eds M A Gatzoulis, G D Webb & P Daubeney). Elsevier, Philadelphia.

Nieminen HP, Jokinen EV & Sairanen HI (2001) Late results of pediatric cardiac surgery in Finland – a population based study with 96% follow-up. *Circulation*, **104**, 570–575.

Nollert G, Fischlein T, Bouterwek S, *et al.* (1997) Long-term survival in patients with repair of tetralogy of Fallot: 36-year follow-up of 490 survivors of the first year after surgical repair. *Journal of the American College of Cardiology*, **30**, 1374–1383.

Vonder-Muhll I, Cumming G & Gatzoulis MA (2003) Risky business: insuring adults with congenital heart disease. *European Heart Journal*, **25**, 1595–1600.

Travel and driving

Anon (1996) Assessment of the cardiac patient for fitness to drive: 1996 update. *Canadian Journal of Cardiology*, **12**, 1164–1170.

Antiplatelet Trialist's Collaboration (1994) Collaborative overview of randomized trials of antiplatelet therapy III. Reduction in venous thrombosis and pulmonary embolism by antiplatelet prophylaxis against surgical and medical patients. *British Medical Journal*, **308**, 235–246.

Blitzer ML, Saliba BC, Ghantous AE, Marieb MA & Schoenfeld MH (2003) Causes of impaired consciousness while driving a motorized vehicle. *American Journal of Cardiology*, **91**, 1373–1374.

Durmowicz AG (2001) Pulmonary edema in 6 children with Down syndrome during travel to moderate altitude. *Pediatrics*, **108**, 443–447.

Epstein AE, Miles WM, Benditt DG, *et al.* (1996) Personal and public safety issues related to arrhythmias that may affect consciousness: implications for regulation and physician recommendations. *Circulation*, **94**, 1147–1166.

Harnick E, Hutter PA, Hoorntje TM, *et al.* (1996) Air travel and adults with cyanotic congenital heart disease. *Circulation*, **93**, 273–276.

Herner B, Smedby B & Ysander L (1966) Sudden illness as a cause of motor vehicle accidents. *British Journal of Internal Medicine*, **23**, 37–41.

Jung W, Anderson M, Camm AJ, *et al.* (1997) Recommendations for driving of patients with implantable cardioverter defibrillators. *European Heart Journal*, **18**, 1210–1219.

Pulmonary Embolism Prevention (PEP) Trial Collaborative Group (2000) Prevention of pulmonary embolism and deep vein thrombosis with low dose aspirin: the Pulmonary Embolism Prevention (PEP) trial. *Lancet*, **355**, 1295–1302.

Scurr JH, Machin SJ, Bailey-King S, Mackie IJ, McDonald S & Smith PD (2001) Frequency and prevention of symptomless deep-vein thrombosis in long-haul flights: a randomized trial. *Lancet*, **357**, 1485–1489.

Task Force Report (1998) Driving and heart disease. *European Heart Journal*, **19**, 1165–1177.

CHAPTER 7

Long-Term Outcome

There has been a marked improvement in the pediatric mortality data for congenital lesions over the last 60 years (see Table 7.1). This has primarily been due to improved surgical techniques. Improving on the mortality rates due to progressive decline in cardiac function or pulmonary vascular disease are the equivalent 21st-century challenges. As new generations of patients with very complex lesions reach adulthood, mortality in adulthood may actually increase. For example, the first patients with hypoplastic left heart syndrome are now reaching adult practitioners.

At present, only the simplest cardiac defects are associated with a normal long-term survival. Even simple lesions like secundum atrial septal defects(ASDs) and coarctation reduce life expectancy. Unfortunately, unlike the pediatric population, detailed figures are unavailable regarding lifelong outcome. There is to date no effective risk stratification for these adult groups.

Lesions thought to be associated with poor outcome in adults

• Anything to do with ventricular dysfunction!
• Univentricular hearts: repaired and unrepaired.
• Cyanotic lesions.
• Pulmonary hypertension.
• Shone's syndrome, especially if multiple procedures.
• Pulmonary atresia with ventricular septal defect (VSD) and aortopulmonary collaterals.

Figure 7.1 illustrates congenital heart disease (CHD) mortality in the UK in 2001.

Table 7.1 Incidence of congenital lesions and outcomes in the UK

	Birth year	No. born with CHD	Survival at 1 year	Survival at 18 years
Complex lesions	1940–60	24,930	20%	10%
	1960–80	25,890	50%	35%
	1980–90	11,325*	70%	50%
Simple lesions	1940–60	74,790	90%	90%
	1960–80	77,680	90%	90%
	1980–90	33,980*	90%	90%

*Reflects fall in total birth rate; no change in % of live births affected.

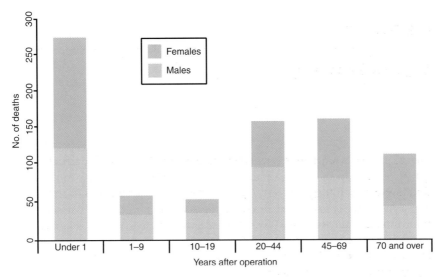

Fig. 7.1 Total numbers of deaths from congenital heart disease in the UK in 2001 (categorized by age at the time of death).

Transplantation

Cardiac transplantation with or without lung transplantation offers a second chance for congenital patients with failing hearts. However, this is not a panacea and is reserved for those who will gain symptomatic, as well as prognostic, benefit.

The barriers to transplantation are as for the non-congenital groups, with organ shortage being the most important. However, congenital patients have added difficulties. These include an increased incidence of hepatitis B and C from childhood transfusions; previous sternotomies and thoracotomies; abnormal venous connections requiring extra tissue at the time of the transplant and clotting disorders (especially if cyanosed). Indeed, outcome has been guarded for certain lesions, such that centers may be reluctant to accept particular patient groups for transplantation, for example, patients with pulmonary atresia and a VSD (also called tetralogy with pulmonary atresia and multiple aortic-to-pulmonary artery collaterals—MAPCAs; see Chapter 16). These patients have multiple aortopulmonary collaterals which cause excessive bleeding at the time of surgery. At present patients with congenital heart disease comprise about 1% of adult heart transplants.

Heart or heart–lung transplantation

The crucial issue here is the degree of pulmonary vascular disease, if present. Pulmonary pressures and pulmonary vascular resistance should always be assessed, including a full reversibility study (e.g. using high flow oxygen, nitric oxide, sodium nitroprusside) before scheduling surgery. Most transplantation units will not support lone heart transplantation if the trans-pulmonary gradient (mean pulmonary artery pressure minus the mean pulmonary wedge pressure) is 15 mmHg or greater. Other units use pulmonary resistance measurements (needs to be less than 6 Wood units at rest or 3 with maximal vasodilation). The outcome for heart–lung transplant is less encouraging than that for heart transplantation alone (a 5-year survival of 36% compared to 60% in heart transplantation alone). Other options include a single lung transplant in combination with an intracardiac repair.

Assist devices

With the limitation in organ availability, transplantation is unlikely to be the answer for the failing adult congenital patient at least in the next decade. There is therefore a gap in our treatment options that may be filled by intra-aortic balloon pumps in the short term and assist devices/mechanical hearts in the long term. There is, at present, limited experience in this group of patients with regard to left ventricular or biventricular assist devices, either as a bridge to transplantation or as destination therapy.

Palliative care

Unfortunately, several of the most severe forms of congenital heart disease are associated with marked shortening of life expectancy. In this setting, it is hoped that improving surgical techniques and newer treatment modalities (such as automatic implantable cardiac defibrillators; AICDs) will go some way to improve long-term outcomes.

However, for a subgroup of patients there are limited options. Although one-third of deaths occur suddenly, other patients deteriorate over a period of months or even years. In this scenario it is helpful, if possible, to have discussed end-of-life issues such as resuscitation and to have the patient's wishes documented. This potentially lessens the pain for family members who may need to make treatment decisions at a time of great stress and upset.

Heart failure nurse specialists and/or palliative care teams may be helpful in improving symptom control and smoothing the 'hospital–home' interface for patients. Being able to remain at home with support is very important for many patients and is something cardiologists can learn from their oncology/palliative care colleagues. Patient help groups and bereavement support groups are very helpful resources for a family coming to terms with the critical nature of their relative's illness.

Symptoms in terminal cardiac disease

- Breathlessness (may respond to home oxygen therapy).
- Anxiety (small doses of benzodiazepines, opiates; treat depression).
- Anorexia (treat right heart failure; steroids may increase fluid retention).
- Cachexia.
- Profound lethargy.
- Syncope (exclude treatable rhythm disturbances).
- Refractory edema (home administration of intravenous diuretic).
- Abdominal distension (as above).

Further reading

Hanratty B, Hibbert D, Mair F, *et al.* (2002) Doctors' perceptions of palliative care for heart failure: focus group study. *British Medical Journal*, **325**, 581–585.

Petersen S, Peto V & Rayner M (2003) *Congenital heart disease statistics 2003*. British Heart Foundation Health Promotion Research Group, University of Oxford.

Pigula FA, Gandhi SK, Ristich J, *et al.* (2001) Cardiopulmonary transplantation for congenital heart disease in the adult. *Journal of Heart and Lung Transplantation*, **20**(3), 297–303.

PART 2

Common Lesions

CHAPTER 8

Atrial Septal Defects and Anomalous Pulmonary Venous Drainage

Atrial septal defect

Description of the lesion

An atrial septal defect (ASD) is a direct communication between the cavities of the atrial chambers, which permits shunting of blood. In the normal heart, the true atrial septum is within the rims of the oval fossa, the majority of the remaining tissue separating the atrial chambers being composed of an infolding of the atrial wall. The morphology of the various types of ASDs is shown in Fig. 8.1.

Secundum ASDs—defects of the oval fossa—are by far the most common. A *superior sinus venosus ASD* occurs when there is a deficiency of infolding of the atrial wall in the environs of the superior vena cava (SVC). It is overridden by the mouth of the SVC, which in turn has a biatrial connection. Most frequently, the pulmonary veins from part of the right lung are also involved, connecting anomalously to the SVC near to its junction with the atria. *Inferior sinus*

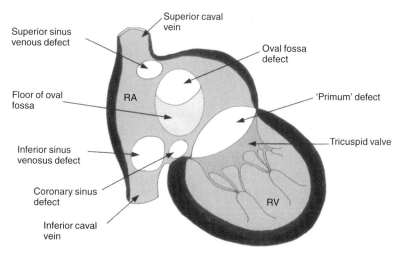

Fig. 8.1 Various types of ASD as seen from the right side of the heart. RA, right atrium; RV, right ventricle.

venosus ASDs overriding the inferior vena cava (IVC) are much less common. The rarest type of ASD is a deficiency of the party wall between the coronary sinus and the left atrium, producing an interatrial communication through the mouth of the coronary sinus, a so-called *coronary sinus ASD. Primum ASDs* or *partial atrioventricular septal defects (AVSD)* will be discussed in Chapter 10. Large intra-atrial communications may represent a confluence of one type of ASD with another.

The size of the ASD and the relative compliance of the right ventricle and the pulmonary vascular bed (in relationship to the left ventricle) determine the degree of intra-atrial shunting (left to right under normal circumstances for the vast majority of isolated ASDs).

Associated lesions

When ASD is the primary diagnosis, associated malformations occur in about 30% of cases.
- Partial anomalous pulmonary venous connection (almost universal with superior sinus venosus ASDs, less common with secundum ASDs and rare with primum ASDs).
- Pulmonary valve stenosis.
- Mitral stenosis or mitral valve prolapse.
- Ventricular septal defect.
- Patent ductus arteriosus.
- Coarctation of the aorta.

Incidence and etiology

- One of the most common congenital heart disease (CHD) defects as an isolated lesion, occurring in about 6–10% of all cardiac malformations.
- ASD and a bicuspid aortic valve are the two most common CHD defects presenting in adulthood.
- More common in females (2:1).
- There is a well-recognized association of ASD with Down syndrome (secundum or primum), with Holt Oram syndrome (secundum, see glossary) and occasionally as a familial occurrence (secundum, associated with delayed atrioventricular conduction).
- Secundum defects are the most common (60%), with primum defects accounting for 20% and superior sinus venosus defects 15%. The other types are rare.

Presentation and course in childhood

- Most children with an ASD present with a murmur and are asymptomatic.
- Occasionally, infants may present with breathlessness, recurrent chest infections and even heart failure.
- In the current era, many children are referred to a pediatric cardiologist for spurious reasons and found to have an atrial septal defect on echocardiographic testing.

• Children with sizeable ASDs and right heart dilatation should undergo elective closure of their defect for prognostic reasons during the first decade of life, irrespective of symptoms.

Course in adulthood

• Most adults present with symptoms usually in the third or fourth decade of life. These are usually breathlessness on exertion and/or palpitations due to atrial tachyarrhythmias. This often correlates with an increase in left-to-right shunting seen with increasing age.

• Occasionally, adults may present with cardiac enlargement on routine chest radiograph or a heart murmur. The latter type of presentation is particularly common among pregnant women, due to enhanced clinical signs (more obvious flow murmur and fixed splitting of the second heart sound) reflecting increased circulating plasma volume.

• Adults with ASDs have reduced survival if ASD closure takes place after the age of 25 years. Other late complications of unrepaired ASDs are right heart failure, recurrent pneumonia and pulmonary hypertension, atrial flutter and fibrillation and paradoxical embolus and stroke.

Examination

The *diagnostic work-up* should:
• document the ASD, its type and size;
• determine its hemodynamic effects:
  – presence and degree of right atrial and ventricular dilatation,
  – status of right ventricular function,
  – shunt magnitude,
  – pulmonary arterial pressure;
• determine the presence of associated anomalies that need to be addressed; and
• establish whether there is a history of sustained arrhythmia that required arrhythmia intervention at the time of ASD closure.

It should include a detailed *history* and *clinical examination*:
• right ventricular left parasternal impulse;
• wide and fixed splitting of the second heart sound: cardinal physical sign of an ASD, not always present;
• pulmonary ejection systolic murmur at the upper left sternal edge;
• tricuspid mid-diastolic murmur at the lower left sternal edge, which may radiate towards the cardiac apex;
• accentuated pulmonary component of the second heart sound, suggesting raised pulmonary arterial pressure;
• cyanosis; uncommon, more likely with a large defect or virtually common atrium, an inferior sinus venosus defect, a large coronary sinus defect, with pulmonary vascular disease, or associated pulmonary stenosis, right ventricular dysfunction or Ebstein's malformation.

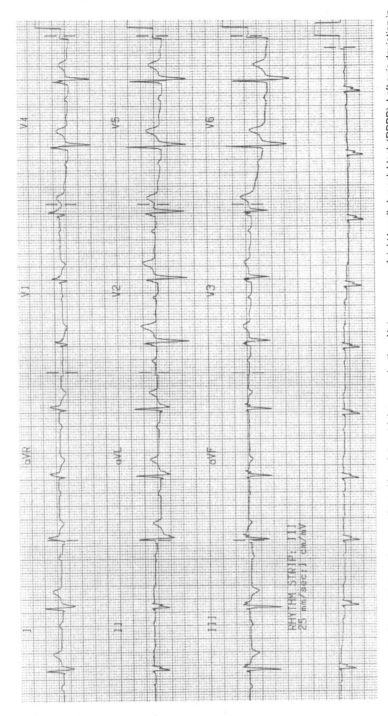

Fig. 8.2 12-lead electrocardiogram from a patient with an intra-atrial communication. Note presence of right bundle branch block (RBBB). Left axis deviation in keeping with a primum ASD (95% of patients with a primum ASD have a superior axis, i.e. extreme right or left axis deviation). Absence of RVH suggesting no pulmonary hypertension. Note normal P wave axis (0–60°) making a high sinus venosus ASD unlikely. 1° heart block (common with primum ASD).

Useful investigations

- **Pulse oximetry**: normal oxygen saturations are expected.
- **EKG** (see Fig. 8.2)
  - Right axis deviation and incomplete right bundle branch block pattern are common.
  - Evidence of right ventricular hypertrophy, and lengthening of PR interval may be present.
  - Large P waves, suggesting atrial overload.
- **Chest radiography** in adults with significant ASDs reveals:
  - cardiac enlargement with retrosternal filling in the lateral film
  - right atrial dilatation
  - prominent central pulmonary arteries and pulmonary vascular markings.
- **Echocardiography** (see Fig. 8.3)
  - The diagnosis is usually confirmed by cross-sectional echocardiography, using a combination of subcostal and parasternal four-chamber sections with colour flow Doppler interrogation.
  - The most important finding is an enlarged right ventricle which might be the only clue to an ASD in the adult with a poor window.
  - The presence of tricuspid regurgitation will permit a Doppler estimate of pulmonary artery pressure.

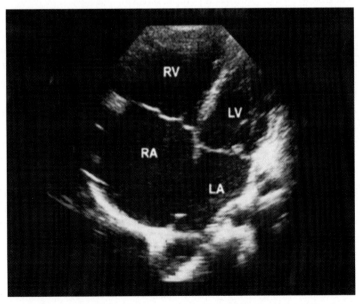

Fig. 8.3 Transthoracic echocardiogram from patient with a large secundum ASD. Note massive dilatation of the right atrium (RA) and right ventricle (RV) with an echo drop-out at the level of ASD and a squashed left ventricle (LV). Smaller ASDs can be missed with transthoracic echocardiography. If right heart dilatation is present, transesophageal imaging may be necessary. LA, left atrium.

 – A high index of suspicion is sometimes required to make the correct diagnosis and transesophageal studies are often needed in the adult patient to establish the site and size of the defect and the connection of the pulmonary veins.
 – Three-dimensional and intracardiac echocardiogram may also have a role.

Management options for adults with ASD

The management of the adult with an ASD is primarily determined by the size and type of the defect, associated lesions and the presence and degree of pulmonary vascular resistance. Currently, *indications for ASD closure* are as follows:
• Presence of an ASD with cardiac enlargement on the chest radiography, a dilated right ventricle on an echocardiogram and a pulmonary artery systolic or mean pressure 50% or less than the corresponding aortic pressures. *This is irrespective of symptoms (many of these patients have symptoms such as exercise intolerance without being aware of it).* Patients should be considered for elective closure irrespective of age provided there are no specific contraindications (see below). Younger and older patients would benefit from ASD closure compared to medical therapy in terms of:
 – survival;
 – functional class;
 – exercise tolerance;
 – reduction of risk of heart failure; and
 – reduction of risk of pulmonary hypertension; *however,*
 – patients older than 40 years of age and particularly those with preoperative rhythm disturbance remain at risk of sustained atrial arrhythmia after closure. *For the latter group, consideration should be given to arrhythmia targeted intervention either via transcatheter techniques, with new mapping and ablative systems or surgical atrial ablative procedures.*
• History of cryptogenic TIA or stroke in the presence of an ASD or persistent foramen ovale and right-to-left shunting demonstrated on contrast echocardiogram.
Contraindications for closure include a pulmonary vascular resistance of more than 7–8 units or a defect diameter of less than 8 mm (with no evidence of right heart dilatation) in a patient who is symptom-free.

All *secundum defects* should be considered for transcatheter closure with one of the various devices that are available. Defects up to 40 mm in diameter can be closed with the Amplatzer® septal occluder, usually resulting in improvement in symptoms at any age. Very large oval fossa defects and other types can be closed only by surgery using cardiopulmonary bypass with the potential for greater morbidity in the elderly with arrhythmias. Minimally invasive surgery is also an alternative for selected patients.

Device closure

Figure 8.4 shows the sequence of device closure.
• Early and intermediate follow-up is excellent after device closure.

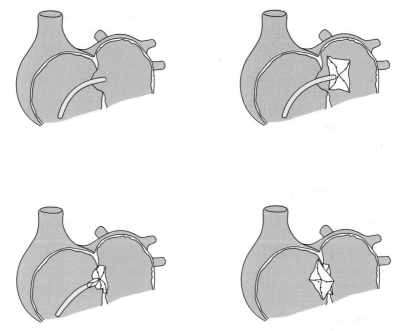

Fig. 8.4 Transcatheter closure of a secundum ASD. Catheter introduced from the right atrium through the defect to the left atrium (top left panel). Distal part of the device released (top right panel). Device and introducer are pulled back with the former opposing against the left atrial aspect of the intra-atrial wall (bottom left panel). Finally, proximal part of the device is released and deployed (bottom right panel).

• The intermediate results are comparable to surgery with a high rate of shunt closure and few major complications.
• As with the surgical group, functional capacity improves and supraventricular arrhythmias are better tolerated and more responsive to medical management.
• Occasionally, residual atrial septal defects are encountered either after catheter or surgical closure. Unless responsible for a significant left-to-right shunt (i.e. large residual ASDs) generally they do not require additional intervention.
• Longer follow-up is needed to determine the incidence of arrhythmias and thromboembolic complications late after device closure.

Surgical outcomes
• Secundum ASDs without pulmonary hypertension should undergo surgical closure with a very low (<1%) operative mortality.
• Early and long-term follow-up is excellent. Preoperative symptoms, if any, should decrease or abate.

• Pre-existing atrial flutter and fibrillation may persist unless concomitant arrhythmia targeting procedures are performed. Likewise, atrial flutter and/or fibrillation may arise de novo after repair in the older patient, but are better tolerated and often more responsive to antiarrhythmic therapy.

Medical management
This is primarily the management of the associated complications of right heart failure, atrial tachyarrhythmia and occasionally pulmonary hypertension (see management of patients with Eisenmenger physiology), when present.

Endocarditis recommendations
Endocarditis prophylaxis is only needed for primum defects and patients with valvular regurgitation or other associated lesions. Endocarditis prophylaxis is also advised for patients undergoing catheter closure for a period of 6 months.

Exercise
Most adults are in New York Heart Association functional class 1 or 2 and require no limitation on their permitted exercise.

Pregnancy and contraception
Pregnancy is well tolerated by most women with an unoperated atrial septal defect. Cardiological review is recommended because of the small risk of paradoxical embolus and stroke, arrhythmia and heart failure. If circumstances allow, ASDs should be closed prior to pregnancy. However, pregnancy can usually be allowed to continue. For a secundum defect, transcatheter device closure can be performed during pregnancy (with transesophageal or intracardiac echocardiography). The only contraindication to pregnancy in women with ASDs, *operated or not*, is persisting pulmonary hypertension.

Late complications
• Premature death
• Right heart failure
• Left ventricular dysfunction
• Tricuspid and mitral valve regurgitation
• Atrial flutter/fibrillation
• Sinus node dysfunction
• Paradoxical thromboembolism
• Endocarditis (rare)
• Systemic arterial hypertension
• Pulmonary hypertension/pulmonary vascular disease (usually a very late complication)

Key clinical points

- ASDs with right heart dilatation merit elective closure for symptomatic improvement and prognostication irrespective of age.
- Catheter closure is preferable and indeed possible for the majority of secundum ASDs.
- Atrial tachyarrhythmias are likely to persist or develop following late ASD closure. Arrhythmia targeting intervention should be considered at the time of ASD closure. Prophylactic anticoagulation for 6 months after closure is recommended for the older patient, while right heart and pulmonary venous remodeling takes place (Fig. 8.5).

Further reading

Attie F, Rosas M, Granados N, Buendia A, Zabal C, Calderon J (2001) Anatomical closure for secundum atrial septal defect in patients aged over 40 years. A randomised clinical trial. *Journal of the American College of Cardiology*, **38**(7), 2035–2042.

Brochu M-C, Baril J-F, Dore A, Juneau M, De Guise P, Mercier L-A (2002) Improvement in exercise capacity in asymptomatic and mildly symptomatic adults after atrial septal defect percutaneous closure. *Circulation*, **106**, 1821–1826.

Gatzoulis MA, Freeman MA, Siu SC, Webb GD, Harris L (1999) Atrial arrhythmia after surgical closure of atrial septal defects in adults. *New England Journal of Medicine*, **40**, 839–846.

Kobayashi J, Yamamoto F, Nakano K, Sasako Y, Kitamura S, Kosakai Y (1998) Maze procedure for atrial fibrillation associated with atrial septal defect. *Circulation*, **98**, 399–402.

Murphy J, Gersh B, McGoon M, *et al.* (1999) Long-term outcome after surgical repair of isolated atrial septal defect. *New England Journal of Medicine*, **323**, 1645–1650.

Rigby M (1999) The era of transcatheter closure of atrial septal defects. *Heart*, **81**, 227–228.

St John Sutton M, Tajik A, McGoon D (1981) Atrial septal defects in patients aged 60 years or older: operative results and long-term postoperative followup. *Circulation*, **64**, 402–409.

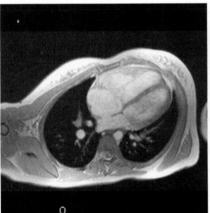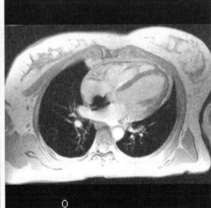

Fig. 8.5 Cardiac magnetic resonance imaging (MRI) showing right heart remodeling following closure of a secundum ASD with an Amplatzer® device. Interval between the baseline and the post-ASD closure MRI of 6 months. The magnitude of reduction in right heart dilatation is inversely related to age and leads to improved left ventricular filling, increased cardiac output and better exercise capacity.

Partial anomalous pulmonary venous drainage

Description of the lesion

Partial anomalous pulmonary venous drainage (PAPVD) is defined as at least one pulmonary vein connected to the right (rather than the left) atrium. The connection can be directly to the right atrium or indirectly via either the (superior or inferior) vena cava. The most common variant of PAPVD is the anomalous connection of right pulmonary vein/s to the superior vena cava or the right atrium. Anomalous pulmonary venous drainage from the left lung is less common, usually to the left brachiocephalic vein or to the coronary sinus.

Scimitar syndrome

The scimitar syndrome constitutes a specific entity characterized by:
• PAPVD of the right pulmonary vein/s to the inferior vena cava;
• anomalous systemic arterial supply to the right lung; and
• variable degree of right lung hypoplasia with or without pulmonary sequestration.

Associated lesions

The most frequently lesion associated with PAPVD is an atrial septal defect. PAPVD is extremely common in sinus venosus defects (particularly superior) and is seen in approximately 2% of patients with secundum defects. Other associated lesions which may occur with PAPVD are congenital mitral stenosis or atresia, tetralogy of Fallot, ventricular septal defect, coarctation of the aorta, patent ductus arteriosus, aortic stenosis and hypoplasia of the aorta.

Genetics/epidemiology

Partial anomalous pulmonary venous connection is a rare congenital lesion (between 0.4 and 0.7% in an autopsy series). Risk of recurrence is small.

Presentation in childhood and adulthood

Patients with isolated PAPVD are usually asymptomatic early in life. Patients who develop symptoms usually have more than one anomalously draining pulmonary vein and/or associated lesions. Symptoms resemble those of patients with an atrial septal defect, namely exertional dyspnea, atrial tachyarrhyrhmia and later on in the course of the disease right heart failure and pulmonary hypertension.

Early development of pulmonary hypertension during childhood—although rare—has been reported in patients with or without an atrial septal defect and in patients with scimitar syndrome, and carries a poorer prognosis.

Examination

The *diagnostic work-up* should document:

• PAPVD;
• the presence or not of right heart dilatation;

- the presence of associated intracardiac lesions; and
- the degree of pulmonary hypertension, if present.

Seek the following signs on *clinical examination*:

- right ventricular left parasternal impulse;
- wide and fixed splitting of the second heart sound, not always present;
- tricuspid mid-diastolic murmur at the lower left sternal edge, which might radiate towards the cardiac apex;
- accentuated pulmonary component of the second heart sound, suggesting raised pulmonary arterial pressure.

Useful investigations

- **EKG**:
  - right bundle branch block pattern is common;
  - right axis deviation may present if right heart dilation is present;
  - first-degree heart block is common with significant PAPVD.
- **Chest radiography**:
  - right heart dilatation in the lateral film;
  - dilatation of central pulmonary arteries;
  - increased pulmonary vascular markings are common;
  - signs of pulmonary hypertension may be present.
- **Echocardiography**:
  - right atrial/ventricular dilation in the four-chamber and long parasternal axis views (in patients with a significant PAPVD);
  - transesophageal echocardiography may assist in documenting the site of drainage of the PAPVDs;
  - pulse-wave Doppler would exclude stenoses at the anastomotic site for those who have undergone repair (uncommon).
- **Cardiac MRI** (with MR angiography): assist in the delineation of origin, course and anastomotic site of the anomalous vein(s).
- **Cardiac catheterization**: should be employed when pulmonary hypertension is suspected or for patients older than 40 years of age referred for surgery (to exclude coexisting coronary artery disease).

PAPVD closure in adulthood should be considered in the presence of right heart dilatation, irrespective of age and presence of symptoms. Patients with established arrhythmia—atrial flutter in particular—should be considered for concomitant arrhythmia intervention at the time of surgery.

Pregnancy

Pregnancy in operated patients should be tolerated well in the absence of pulmonary hypertension. Patients who have undergone late repair may have persisting right atrial dilatation and be at risk of atrial arrhythmia.

Level of follow-up

Provided that there is no residual pulmonary hypertension, and important stenoses of pulmonary and systemic venous channels have been ruled out, patients do not require tertiary follow-up. Patients who have undergone late repair should be alerted about the risk of late atrial flutter and/or fibrillation and/or bradycardia.

Endocarditis prophylaxis

Patients with unoperated PAPVD require endocarditis prophylaxis when associated lesions, such as tricuspid regurgitation, are present.

Exercise

Patients with repaired PAPVD need no exercise restrictions, with the exception of those with pulmonary hypertension and or exercise-induced atrial tachyarrhythmia.

Scimitar syndrome

Associated lesions are common in scimitar syndrome (in 25% of patients, especially atrial and ventricular septal defects, patent ductus arteriosus, coarctation of the aorta, and tetralogy of Fallot).

Scimitar syndrome is a rare condition with low recurrence rate.

Presentation

• Coincidental finding on chest radiography; heart in middle or dextro-position, due to right lung hypoplasia with scimitar vein.
• Heart murmur, due to associated lesions.
• Exertional dyspnea and/or palpitations, depending on the degree of the hemodynamic abnormalities involved.
• Frequent pulmonary infections with or without hemoptysis, due to lung sequestration.

Examination

• Cardiac apex may be displaced to the right (secondary to right lung hypoplasia).
• Signs of associated defects (ASD or VSD) may be present.
• Signs of right heart dilatation and/or pulmonary hypertension may be present (as per ASD patients).

Useful investigations

• **Chest radiography**:
  – degree of right lung hypoplasia (Fig. 8.6);
  – presence of the scimitar vein;
  – dilatation of central pulmonary arteries may be present (usually with associated intracardiac defects);
  – increased pulmonary vascular markings or signs of pulmonary hypertension may be present.

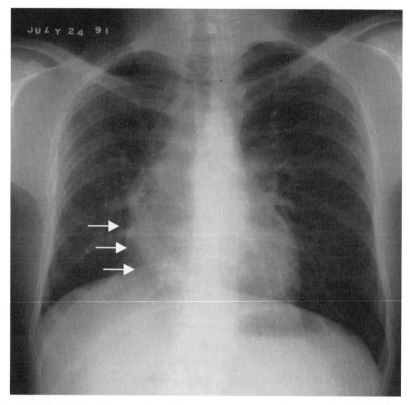

Fig. 8.6 Patient with scimitar syndrome following repair. Note persisting right lung hypoplasia (with secondary right heart displacement), dilated central pulmonary arteries in keeping with the previous large left-to-right shunt (patient had also a large secundum ASD, now repaired) and the ectatic scimitar vein previously draining to the IVC to RA junction. IVC, inferior vena cava; RA, right atrium.

- **Echocardiography**:
  - defines intracardiac anatomy;
  - demonstrates pulmonary venous return;
  - delineates hemodynamics and the need for intervention;
  - when tricuspid regurgitation is present, it assists in estimation of right ventricular and pulmonary arterial pressure.
- **Cardiac MRI** (with MR angiography): assists greatly in delineating the scimitar vein and the anomalous arterial lung supply from the aorta.
- **Spiral CT**: provides additional information on pulmonary pathology (sequestration, bleeding or bronchiectasis).
- **Cardiac catheterization**: should be employed when pulmonary hypertension is suspected, or for patients older than 40 years of age referred for surgery.

Repair of the scimitar syndrome should be guided by the direct hemodynamic effects of the anomalous pulmonary venous return and the effects of associated lesions. The same principles as with ASD and PAPVD should apply.

Additional indication for cardiothoracic intervention may exist in patients with recurrent respiratory infections and/or hemoptysis, and this needs to be assessed in conjunction with respiratory physicians and thoracic surgeons. Such patients with severe sequestration of the lung and recurrent pulmonary infections may benefit from resection of the sequestrated lung and ligation or catheter occlusion of the anomalous arterial blood supply to respective lung segment(s).

Pregnancy
Pregnancy in operated patients should be tolerated well in the absence of pulmonary hypertension.

Level of follow-up
Patients with scimitar syndrome should remain under periodic tertiary care follow-up.

Endocarditis prophylaxis
Patients require lifelong endocarditis prophylaxis when valvular regurgitation or associated lesions, other than an ASD, are present.

Exercise
Patients with repaired scimitar syndrome, in general, need no exercise restrictions.

Late complications of PAPVD and scimitar syndrome
(In patients with significant left-to-right shunts and right heart dilatation):
• reduced lifespan;
• right heart failure;
• atrial flutter/fibrillation;
• sinus node disease;
• endocarditis (very rare);
• pulmonary hypertension/pulmonary vascular disease (may occur earlier than in patients with ASD alone);
• recurrent pulmonary infections and or hemoptysis in patients with the Scimitar syndrome

Key clinical points

• All patients with PAPVD or the scimitar syndrome with left-to-right shunting and right heart dilatation merit consideration for repair for symptomatic improvement and prognostication.
• This should be done irrespective of the presence of overt symptoms and age of the patient.

- Pulmonary hypertension may develop in patients with PAPVD or scimitar syndrome earlier than in those with an ASD (for reasons which are not clear), hence repair should not be delayed when indications for intervention are present.
- Patients with scimitar syndrome may need thoracic surgery for pulmonary complications, and this needs to be addressed in conjunction to their hemodynamics relating to the cardiac defect(s).
- Follow-up is advisable for patients with any degree of pulmonary hypertension and all patients with the scimitar syndrome.

Further reading

Mathey J, Galey JJ, Logeais Y, *et al*. (1968) Anomalous pulmonary venous return into inferior vena cava and associated bronchovascular anomalies (the scimitar syndrome). Report of three cases and review of the literature. *Thorax,* **23**, 398–407.

Prasad SK, Soukias N, Hornung T, Pennell DJ, Gatzoulis MA, Mohiaddin RH (2004) Role of MRA in the diagnosis of multiple aorto-pulmonary collateral arteries and partial anomalous pulmonary venous drainage. *Circulation,* **109**(2), 207–214.

Saalouke MG, Shapiro SR, Perry LW (1977) Isolated partial anomalous pulmonary venous drainage associated with pulmonary vascular obstructive disease. *American Journal of Cardiology,* **39**, 439–444.

Smallhorn JF, Pauperio H, Benson LM, Rowe RD (1985) Pulsed Doppler assessment of pulmonary vein obstruction. *American Heart Journal,* **110**, 483–486.

Vogel M, Berger F, Kramer A, Alexi-Meskishvili V, Lange PE (1999) Incidence of secondary pulmonary hypertension in adults with atrial septal or sinus venosus defect. *Heart,* **82**, 30–33.

CHAPTER 9

Ventricular Septal Defect

Description of the lesion

The ventricular septum is composed of a muscular septum that can be divided into three major components (inlet, trabecular and outlet) and a small membranous septum lying just underneath the aortic valve. Ventricular septal defects (VSDs) are classified into three main categories according to their location and margins (see Fig. 9.1).

- *Muscular VSD*: bordered entirely by myocardium; trabecular, inlet or outlet in location.
- *Membranous VSD*: often with inlet, outlet or trabecular extension and bordered in part by fibrous continuity between the leaflets of an atrioventricular valve and an arterial valve.
- *Doubly committed subarterial VSD*: situated in the outlet septum and bordered by fibrous continuity of the aortic and pulmonary valves.

Incidence

Ventricular septal defects are one of the most common congenital malforma-

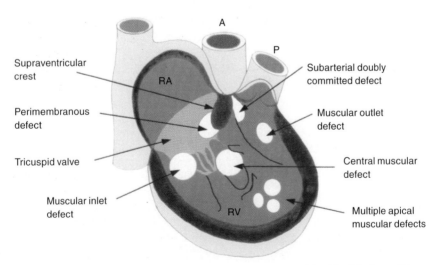

Fig. 9.1 Various types of ventricular septal defect as seen from the right side of the heart. RA, right atrium; RV, right ventricle; A, aorta; P, pulmonary artery.

tions of the heart, accounting for approximately 20% of all congenital cardiac malformations.

Presentation and course in childhood

• *A restrictive VSD* is defined as a defect which produces a significant pressure gradient between the left ventricle and the right ventricle, is usually accompanied by a small (<1.5/1.0) shunt and does not cause significant hemodynamic derangement. Spontaneous closure of a perimembranous VSD or of a small muscular VSD during childhood is common. Children are most often asymptomatic.
• *A moderately restrictive VSD* is accompanied by a moderate shunt (Qp/Qs = 1.5–2.5/1.0) and will pose a hemodynamic burden on the left ventricle. Children will present with failure to thrive and congestive heart failure.
• *A* large or *nonrestrictive VSD* (Qp/Qs >2.5/1.0) results initially in left ventricular volume overload early in life with a progressive rise in pulmonary artery pressure in childhood.

Physical examination

• *Small restrictive VSD*: high-frequency holosystolic murmur, usually grade 3–4/6, heard with maximal intensity at the left sternal border in the third or fourth intercostal space.
• *Moderately to large nonrestrictive VSD*: displaced cardiac apex with holosystolic murmur as well as an apical diastolic rumble and third heart sound at the apex from the increased flow through the mitral valve.
• *Eisenmenger VSD*: central cyanosis and clubbing of the nail beds with signs of pulmonary hypertension—a right ventricular heave, palpable and loud P_2, and a right-sided S_4—are typically present. In many patients, a pulmonary ejection click and a soft and scratchy systolic ejection murmur, attributable to dilatation of the pulmonary trunk, and a high-pitched decrescendo diastolic murmur of pulmonary regurgitation (Graham Steell) are audible.

Useful investigations

• **EKG**: the EKG mirrors the size of the shunt and the degree of pulmonary hypertension. *Small restrictive VSDs* usually produce a normal tracing. *Moderate size VSDs* produce a broad notched P wave characteristic of left atrial overload as well as signs of left ventricular volume overload, namely deep Q and tall R waves with tall T waves in lead V_{5-6}. Atrial fibrillation may also be present.
• **Chest radiography**: the chest radiograph reflects the magnitude of the shunt as well as the degree of pulmonary hypertension. A moderate sized shunt causes signs of left ventricular dilatation with some pulmonary plethora.

• **Echocardiography**: transthoracic echocardiography can identify the location, size and hemodynamic consequences of the VSD as well as any associated lesions.
• **Cardiac catheterization**: this may be performed to determine the severity of pulmonary vascular disease and the magnitude of intracardiac shunts.

Surgical management

• Moderately restrictive and nonrestrictive VSDs need timely surgical closure.
• When pulmonary hypertension is present, surgical closure may still be considered if there is any of the following:
  – a net left-to-right shunt of at least 1.5/1.0;
  – pulmonary reactivity when challenged with a pulmonary vasodilator (oxygen, nitric oxide);
  – lung biopsy evidence that pulmonary artery changes are reversible.
• Successful transcatheter device closure of perimembranous or muscular VSDs has recently been reported in highly selected cases where the defect is far away from the aortic valve.

Late complications

• *A restrictive VSD* poses an ongoing and relatively high risk of endocarditis. Perimembranous or outlet VSDs can be associated with progressive aortic valve regurgitation due to aortic cusp(s) prolapse into the defect (Fig. 9.2). Late development of subaortic and subpulmonary stenosis has also been reported.
• *A moderately restrictive VSD*, if left untreated, will lead to left atrial and ventricular dilatation and dysfunction in adulthood as well as a variable increase in pulmonary vascular resistance. Important atrial arrhythmias, and less often ventricular arrhythmias, can occur.
• *A nonrestrictive VSD* will lead to irreversible pulmonary vascular changes and systemic pulmonary pressures, the so-called Eisenmenger syndrome (unless the pulmonary bed is protected by pulmonary stenosis).

Recommended follow-up

• Yearly cardiac evaluation is suggested for patients with associated aortic regurgitation, Eisenmenger patients, and adults with significant atrial or ventricular arrhythmias.
• Cardiac surveillance is also recommended for patients who have undergone late repair of moderate or large defects, which are often associated with left ventricular impairment and elevated pulmonary artery pressure at the time of surgery.
• Maintenance of good dental hygiene and antibiotic prophylaxis in these patients with residual patch leaks is very important.

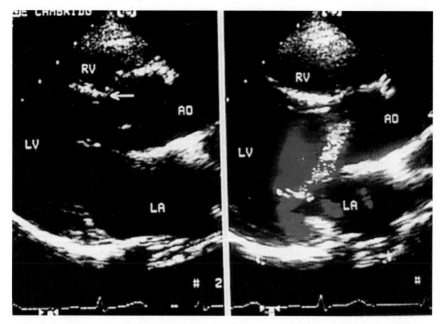

Fig. 9.2 Ventricular septal defect (VSD) with aortic cusp prolapse and secondary aortic regurgitation. Long axis echocardiographic views. Note aortic cusp prolapse into the VSD (arrow, left panel) and aortic regurgitation on color Doppler (right panel). VSD is partially occluded by the protruding cusp. Patient referred for surgery. AO, aorta; LA, left atrium; LV, left ventricle; RV, right ventricle.

• Patients with small restrictive defects need to be seen infrequently.

Endocarditis recommendations
• Subacute bacterial endocarditis prophylaxis is indicated in patients with unrepaired VSD, residual VSD patch leak, associated aortic regurgitation or pulmonary outflow tract obstruction.

Exercise
• Patients with restrictive VSD do not require exercise restrictions.
• Patients with a moderate size VSD and some degree of pulmonary hypertension should limit their exercise to class IA type activities (see Chapter 6).
• Patients with VSD and Eisenmenger physiology should not exercise.

Pregnancy and contraception
• Pregnancy is well tolerated in women with small or moderate VSD and in women with repaired VSD.
• SBE prophylaxis at the time of delivery is indicated in patients with unrepaired VSD or residual VSD patch leak.

• Patients with pulmonary hypertension are at an increased risk during pregnancy and should be assessed on an individual basis.
• Pregnancy is contraindicated in patients with VSD and the Eisenmenger syndrome.

Long-term outcome

• For patients with good to excellent functional class and good left ventricular function prior to surgical closure, life expectancy after surgical correction is close to normal.
• The risk of progressive aortic regurgitation is markedly reduced after surgery, as is the risk of endocarditis, unless a residual VSD persists.
• Intraventricular conduction disturbances are increased after surgical closure and may be responsible for the slight increase in risk of sudden death encountered in this patient population.

Key clinical points

• VSD with Qp/Qs > 2/1 requires surgical closure before irreversible pulmonary hypertension develops.
• Restrictive perimembranous VSD may cause progressive aortic regurgitation and needs careful long-term follow-up.

Further reading

Freed MD (1993) Infective endocarditis in the adult with congenital heart disease. [Review.] *Cardiology Clinics*, **11**, 589–602.

Kidd L, Driscoll DJ, Gersony WM, *et al.* (1993) Second natural history study of congenital heart defects. Results of treatment of patients with ventricular septal defects. *Circulation*, **87**, 38–51.

Neumayer U, Stone S & Somerville J (1998) Small ventricular septal defects in adults. *European Heart Journal*, **19**, 1573–1582. Rhodes LA, Keane JF, Keane JP, *et al.* (1990) Long follow-up (to 43 years) of ventricular septal defect with audible aortic regurgitation. *American Journal of Cardiology*, **66**, 340–345.

Rigby ML & Redington AN (1994) Primary transcatheter umbrella closure of perimembranous ventricular septal defect. *British Heart Journal*, **72**, 368–371.

CHAPTER 10

Atrioventricular Septal Defect

Description of the lesion

Atrioventricular septal defects (AVSDs) comprise a spectrum of anomalies caused by abnormal development of the endocardial cushions which may give rise to partial, intermediate or complete AVSDs (see Fig. 10.1).

• *Partial AVSD*: ostium primum ASD with a 'cleft' left AV valve. The ventricular septum is intact.
• *Intermediate AVSD*: primum ASD with a restrictive VSD and separate, abnormal AV valves.
• *Complete AVSD*: contiguous primum ASD and nonrestrictive VSD, separated only by a common AV valve.

Incidence and etiology

• Most *partial AVSDs* occur in non-Down syndrome patients (>90%).
• Most *complete AVSDs* occur in Down syndrome patients (>75%).
• AVSD may also occur in association with tetralogy of Fallot and other forms of complex congenital heart disease.

Presentation and course in childhood

• *Partial and intermediate AVSD*: patients with partial and intermediate AVSDs have a course similar to that of patients with large secundum ASDs, with the caveat that symptoms may appear sooner when significant mitral regurgitation occurs through the cleft left AV valve. Children are usually asymptomatic or only mildly symptomatic with dyspnea if they have a significant left-to-right shunt and/or if significant 'mitral' regurgitation coexists.
• *Complete AVSD*: most children with complete defects will present with symptoms of congestive heart failure. Down syndrome patients may have already established significant pulmonary hypertension at presentation.

Physical examination

• *Partial AVSD*: systolic ejection murmur with fixed split S$_2$, a prominent left ventricular apex and holosystolic murmur when significant left AV valve regurgitation is present.

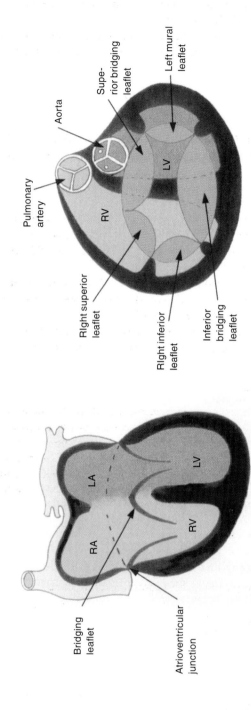

Fig.10.1 Anatomy of atrioventricular septal defect (AVSD). Left panel: note a common atrioventricular junction (universal feature of all AVSDs) and bridging leaflet. Balanced complete AVSD with well-developed right and left ventricles, and both atrial and ventricular communications. Right panel: heart base as seen from above. See five leaflets of a common atrioventricular valve (left mural, superior bridging, right superior, right inferior and inferior bridging leaflet) guarded by a common atrioventricular junction in a patient with a complete AVSD. Patients with partial or incomplete AVSD (also called primum ASD) have fusion of the atrioventricular valve between the superior and inferior bridging leaflets (black central area), producing two separate atrioventricular valves. Note that the left atrioventrioventricular valve has three leaflets as a result. Patients with partial AVSDs have usually only an atrial communication, and occasionally a small but never a large ventricular communication (hence at low risk of developing pulmonary hypertension compared with patients with complete AVSDs). Double dotted line in the center indicates position of the underlying ventricular septum. RA, right atrium; LA, left atrium; RV, right ventricle; LV, left ventricle.

• *Intermediate AVSD*: resembles partial AVSD with the addition of a holosystolic VSD murmur heard best at the left sternal border.
• *Complete AVSD*: a single S_1 (common AV valve), a mid-diastolic murmur from augmented AV valve inflow, and findings of pulmonary hypertension and/or a right-to-left shunt.

Useful investigations

• **EKG**: first-degree AV block (common) and left axis deviation. Partial or complete right bundle branch block is usually associated with right ventricular dilation.
• **Chest radiography**: cardiomegaly and pulmonary plethora are the rule with an enlarged left atrium commonly present.
• **Echocardiography**: echocardiography is essential to document the type of AVSD, assess the magnitude and direction of intracardiac shunting, the degree of AV valve regurgitation, the presence/absence of subaortic stenosis, and to estimate pulmonary artery pressure.
  – The lack of 'offsetting' between the left and right AV valves (the right AV valve being apically displaced in normal hearts) is readily seen in the four-chamber view and is the echo hallmark of AVSD.
• **Cardiac catheterization**: may be performed to determine the severity of pulmonary vascular disease and the magnitude of intracardiac shunts.

Surgical management

Partial AVSD: pericardial patch closure of the primum ASD with concomitant suture (+/– annuloplasty) of the 'cleft' left AV valve should be performed.
Intermediate/complete AVSD: in the absence of irreversible pulmonary hypertension, all patients should undergo surgical repair. The goals of intracardiac repair are ventricular and atrial septation with adequate mitral and tricuspid reconstruction. 'Mitral' valve replacement is sometimes needed when 'mitral' valve repair is not possible.

Late complications

Postoperative complications include:
• recurrent left AV valve regurgitation (most common complication);
• left AV valve stenosis;
• patch dehiscence or residual septal defects;
• development of complete heart block;
• late atrial flutter/fibrillation;
• progressive or de novo subaortic stenosis.

Recommended follow-up

• All patients require long-term follow-up by a cardiologist because of the risk of progressive left AV valve regurgitation (or stenosis), the development of subaortic stenosis, significant atrial arrhythmias, or progression of the commonly present first-degree AV block.

• Particular attention should be paid to those patients with established pulmonary hypertension preoperatively.

Endocarditis recommendations

• SBE prophylaxis is recommended in all patients with unrepaired AVSD.
• SBE prophylaxis is recommended in patients with residual LVOT obstruction, LAVV regurgitation or residual shunt post AVSD repair.

Exercise

• Patients with repaired AVSD and no residual significant hemodynamic lesions have no contraindication to exercise.
• Patients with moderate AVSD shunt and some degree of pulmonary hypertension, moderate to severe residual LVOT obstruction or cardiomegaly should restrain their activities to class IA type (see Chapter 6).
• Patients with AVSD and Eisenmenger physiology should not exercise.

Pregnancy and contraception

• Pregnancy is well tolerated in patients with complete repair and no significant residual lesions.
• Women in NYHA class I and II with unoperated partial AVSD usually tolerate pregnancy very well, but have an increased risk of paradoxical embolization.
• As is the case for VSD, patients with pulmonary hypertension present an increased risk and need specialized advice.

Long-term outcome

• Long-term outcome in patients after surgical correction is relatively good.
• The worst outcome occurs in patients with established pulmonary arterial hypertension preoperatively.
• Recurrent left AV valve regurgitation is the principal cause of late morbidity after surgical repair of AVSDs, necessitating reoperation in at least 10% of patients.
• SBE prophylaxis is needed in most patients after surgical repair due to the persistence of left AV valve regurgitation.

Key clinical points

• Patients with Down syndrome have a propensity to develop pulmonary hypertension at an even earlier age than do other patients with AVSD.
• Recurrent left AV valve regurgitation is the most common complication seen after surgical repair of AVSDs and needs careful follow-up.

Further reading

Bando K, Turrentine MW, Sun K, *et al.* (1995) Surgical management of complete atrioventricular septal defects. A twenty-year experience. *Journal of Thoracic and Cardiovascular Surgery,* **110**, 1543–1552; discussion 1552.

Barnett MG, Chopra PS & Young WP (1988) Long-term follow-up of partial atrioventricular septal defect repair in adults. *Chest,* **94**, 321–324.

Burke RP, Horvath K, Landzberg M, Hyde P, Collins JJ, Jr & Cohn LH (1996) Long-term follow-up after surgical repair of ostium primum atrial septal defects in adults. *Journal of the American College of Cardiology,* **27**, 696–699.

Michielon G, Stellin G, Rizzoli G, *et al.* (1995) Left atrioventricular valve incompetence after repair of common atrioventricular canal defects. *Annals of Thoracic Surgery,* **60**, S604–S609.

CHAPTER 11

Left Ventricular Outflow Tract Disorders

Description of the lesion

Left ventricular outflow tract obstruction (LVOTO) can occur at three levels.

- *Subvalvar LVOTO* can either be discrete (most commonly) or tunnel-shaped.
- *Valvar LVOTO*: a bicuspid aortic valve causing aortic stenosis consists of two cusps, often of unequal size, the larger usually containing a false raphe. *Aortic root enlargement* from cystic medial changes is commonly seen in these patients.
- *Supravalvar LVOTO* may occur rarely in isolation as an hourglass deformity. However, it is more often diffuse, involving other major arteries (pulmonary, coronary and renal arteries) to varying degrees.

Incidence and etiology

- *Subvalvar LVOTO* has a male predominance (2:1). A genetic predisposition has been suggested as there are reports of a familial incidence.
- *Bicuspid aortic valve* (Fig. 11.1) is the most common congenital cardiac anomaly, occurring in 1–2% of the population with a male predominance (4:1).
- *Supravalvar LVOTO* is usually part of Williams syndrome, which is a contiguous gene syndrome associated with neurodevelopmental and multisystem manifestations caused by a deletion at chromosome 7q11.23, but may be familial with normal facies, or associated with rubella syndrome.

Presentation and course in childhood

- *Subvalvar LVOTO* often progresses, but the rate is variable. It is often associated with mild to moderate aortic regurgitation (up to 60% of cases) through an otherwise normal valve that has been damaged by the subvalvar jet of blood. Symptoms vary from none when the obstruction is mild or moderate to dyspnea, chest pain and syncope when the obstruction is severe.
- *Valvar LVOTO* commonly progresses as the patient grows but the rate is variable. Some children will present with aortic stenosis or aortic regurgitation and symptoms will vary from none to mild dyspnea, exertional syncope and/ or chest pain.
- *Supravalvar LVOTO* is usually progressive and aortic regurgitation is common. With Williams syndrome, there are often associated peripheral pulmo-

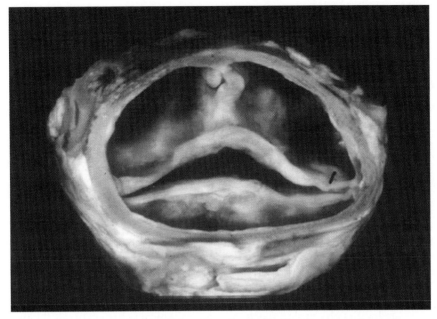

Fig. 11.1 Morphologic specimen of a bicuspid aortic valve. Fusion of two cusps (top part) producing an eccentric functional orifice with the third cusp (bottom part); true bicuspid, i.e. two leaflet aortic valve is uncommon. Note limited opening of the valve with thickening of the cusp edges and failure of complete leaflet coaption, leading to both aortic stenosis and regurgitation.

nary artery or systemic arterial (including coronary ostial) stenoses, which may give rise to chest pain and systemic hypertension.

Physical examination

- *Subvalvar LVOTO*: ejection systolic murmur best heard at the left parasternal border.
- *Bicuspid aortic valve*: ejection systolic click best heard at the apex with either systolic ejection murmur best heard at the second left intercostal space radiating towards the carotids (AS) or diastolic murmur (AR) best heard at the left parasternal border.
- *Supravalvar LVOTO*: ejection systolic murmur best heard at the second left intercostal space, radiating toward the carotids (right > left).

Useful investigations

- **EKG**: the EKG ranges from normal to showing marked left ventricular hypertrophy from severe LVOT obstruction or aortic regurgitation.
- **Chest radiography**: dilatation of the ascending aorta is common with a bicuspid aortic valve (BAV). The left ventricle may be enlarged if severe aortic regurgitation is present.

• **Echocardiography**: this procedure permits identification of the level as well as degree of LVOT obstruction. Assessment of severity of aortic root dilatation and aortic regurgitation can also be performed.

Surgical management

• *Subvalvar LVOTO* should be considered for surgical intervention when a resting catheter gradient or mean echocardiographic gradient is >50 mmHg, symptoms develop, or if combined with progressive aortic regurgitation which is more than mild.
• *Bicuspid aortic valve* requires intervention for:
  – aortic stenosis causing symptoms (dyspnea, angina, presyncope or syncope) or, arguably, 'critical' aortic stenosis (valve area <0.6 cm^2).
  – moderate or severe regurgitation associated with exertional symptoms, or left ventricular end systolic dimensions >55 mm or LVEF <55%.
• Prophylactic surgery for proximal aortic dilatation (>55 mm) is usually recommended.
• Bicuspid aortic stenosis can be treated with balloon valvuloplasty if the valve is non-calcified. Alternatively, significant stenosis or regurgitation can be treated with valve replacement using a mechanical valve, a biological valve or a pulmonary autograft ('Ross procedure'—replacing the aortic valve with the patient's pulmonary valve and implanting a homograft in the pulmonary position).
• *Supravalvar LVOTO* may require surgical intervention for a catheter gradient or mean echocardiographic gradient of >50 mmHg.

Late complications

• *Subvalvar LVOTO*: recurrence of subvalvar LVOTO as well as development of significant aortic regurgitation following repair is not uncommon.
• *Bicuspid aortic valve* stenosis treated by valvuloplasty is associated with progressive recurrent stenosis and/or progressive regurgitation, and may eventually require valve replacement. Aortic root dilatation and dissection also occur.
• In patients with the *Ross procedure*, the pulmonary autograft occasionally deteriorates, giving rise to neo-aortic regurgitation, whereas the pulmonary homograft is expected to stenose with time.
• Recurrence of *supravalvar LVOTO* is uncommon. The long-term durability of the patches or conduits used to relieve the obstruction may be a problem and surveillance should include assessment for aneurysm and endocarditis.

Endocarditis recommendations
• Subacute bacterial endocarditis prophylaxis is recommended in patients with unrepaired LVOT obstruction.

• Subacute bacterial endocarditis prophylaxis is recommended in patients with any residual LVOT obstruction or aortic regurgitaion after surgical repair or balloon dilatation.

• SBE is recommended in any patients with an aortic valve prosthesis.

Exercise

• Patients with mild or no residual LVOT obstruction should have no restriction on physical activities.

• Patients with moderate or severe LVOT obstruction should limit their activities to class IA types (see Chapter 6).

Pregnancy and contraception

LVOTO lesions associated with increased maternal and fetal risk during pregnancy include the following.

• Severe LVOTO with or without symptoms.

• Aortic regurgitation with functional class III to IV.

• LVOTO with moderate or severe LV dysfunction.

• Mechanical prosthetic valves requiring anticoagulation. The latter underscores the importance, when feasible, of valve reconstruction or consideration of a bioprosthesis or pulmonary autograft procedure rather than replacement with a mechanical prosthesis in women having preconception cardiac surgery.

• The presence of bicuspid aortic valve and ascending aortic medial abnormality may predispose to spontaneous aortic dissection in the third trimester.

Recommended follow-up

All patients should have regular cardiology follow-up. Particular attention should be paid to:

• progressive/recurrent stenosis at any level;

• aortic regurgitation;

• ventricular function and/or dilatation;

• aortic root dilatation.

Key clinical points

• Recurrence of *subvalvar LVOTO* is not uncommon, hence the need for lifelong follow-up.

• High prevalence of *aortic root enlargement* in patients with *bicuspid aortic valve* occurs irrespective of altered hemodynamics or age.

• *Supravalvar LVOTO* is often a diffuse disease involving the great arteries as well as pulmonary and coronary arteries.

Further reading

Burks JM, Illes RW, Keating EC & Lubbe WJ (1998) Ascending aortic aneurysm and dissection in young adults with bicuspid aortic valve: implications for echocardiographic surveillance. *Clinical Cardiology*, **21**, 439–443.

Coleman DM, Smallhorn JF, McCrindle BW, Williams WG & Freedom RM. Postoperative follow-up of fibromuscular subaortic stenosis. *Journal of the American College of Cardiology*, **24**, 1558–1564.

Freedom RM, Pelech A, Brand A, *et al.* (1985) The progressive nature of subaortic stenosis in congenital heart disease. *International Journal of Cardiology*, **8**, 137–148.

Niwaya K, Knott-Craig CJ, Lane MM, Chandrasekaren K, Overholt ED & Elkins RC (1999) Cryopreserved homograft valves in the pulmonary position: risk analysis for intermediate-term failure. *Journal of Thoracic and Cardiovascular Surgery*, **117**, 141–146.

Ross D, Jackson M & Davies J (1991) Pulmonary autograft aortic valve replacement: long-term results. *Journal of Cardiac Surgery*, **6**, 529–533.

van Son JA, Schaff HV, Danielson GK, Hagler DJ & Puga FJ (1993) Surgical treatment of discrete and tunnel subaortic stenosis. Late survival and risk of reoperation. *Circulation*, **88**, II159–II169.

Ward C (2000) Clinical significance of the bicuspid aortic valve. *Heart*, **83**, 81–85.

CHAPTER 12

Coarctation of the Aorta

Description of the lesion

Coarctation of the aorta is a stenosis in the aortic arch usually at, or beyond, the site of the duct (Fig. 12.1). In neonates this is often a sling of ductal tissue that causes narrowing of the lumen when the patent ductus arteriosus closes. In adults there is often a more definite obstruction with luminal narrowing distal to the left subclavian artery. Rarely, coarctation can occur at other sites such as the abdominal aorta. Associated vascular abnormalities include hypoplasia of the aortic arch (common) and anomalies of the head and neck vessels including aneurysm formation.

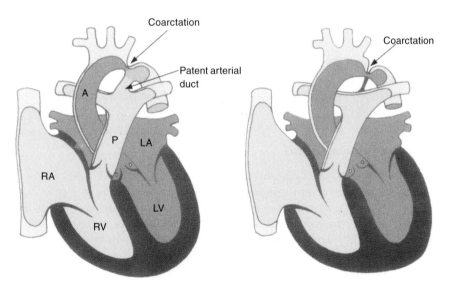

Fig. 12.1 Coarctation of the aorta. Left panel: Coarctation with patent arterial duct, common in neonates. Often patent duct dependent systemic circulation. One of the few pediatric emergencies, with infants presenting with reduced or absent femoral pulses and cardiovascular collapse. Patients require prostaglandin infusion for maintaining patency of the arterial duct until transfer to a cardiothoracic center for prompt coarctation repair.
Right panel: Coarctation with closed arterial duct. Usual pattern in older children or adults (also called native coarctation). Collateral flow is common. Patients often present with either proximal systemic hypertension and/or weak and delayed femoral pulses. RA, right atrium; RV, right ventricle; LA, left atrium; LV, left ventricle; P, pulmonary trunk; A, aorta.

Associated lesions
- Bicuspid aortic valve (with or without aortic stenosis): up to 85%
- Patent arterial ductus, ventricular septal defect
- Bronchial collateral network
- Anomalies of head and neck vessels: 5%
- Intra-cerebral berry aneurysms: 5%
- Proximal arteriopathy (ascending aorta, etc.)
- Multiple left heart obstructive lesions (valvar and subvalvar aortic stenosis, parachute mitral valve—Shone's syndrome)

Incidence and etiology
- 7% of congenital heart lesions
- More common in males (1.5:1)
- A common lesion in Turner syndrome (occurs in up to 25%)
- Rarely—autosomal dominant inheritance

Presentation and course in childhood

The condition often presents in the neonatal period and early childhood depending on the site of the coarctation, the presence of other lesions and the extent to which collaterals are developed.

Neonates usually present with heart failure or 'ductal shock' following closure of the duct. Older children and adults with milder disease come to medical attention with hypertension, murmurs, diminished femoral pulses and occasionally, in adults, acute cardiovascular complications such as cerebrovascular events.

Course in adulthood

The majority of adults with coarctation will already have had surgery. Re-coarctation and aneurysm formation are the commonest repair site complications. Most post-repair adults will be asymptomatic. With increasing age, the incidence of hypertension rises steeply even in the absence of repair site restenosis. By middle age the majority of repaired patients will be hypertensive. Early atherosclerotic disease is common and represents the commonest cause of death in adulthood. Even in the setting of early neonatal repair, life expectancy may not be normal.

Surgical management

Coarctation should be repaired at the time of diagnosis to minimize the long-term adverse sequelae. Surgical repair is by:

• direct end-to-end anastomosis (common in childhood, but interposition graft may be necessary in adulthood);
• subclavian flap repair, arch augmentation using the left subclavian artery (more often in children). Following surgery the left radial pulses may be weak and left arm blood pressure artificially low and unreliable;
• patch grafting (now abandoned due to an increased risk of aneurysm formation);
• long tube grafting or bypass grafting, often needed to deal with long or complex lesions (in adulthood). This includes various forms of anterior grafting with a long conduit from the ascending to the descending intrathoracic aorta running anteriorly over the front of the heart.

Catheter management

Primary stenting is becoming standard treatment for adults with native coarctation or in re-coarctation. This is a relatively safe and highly effective technique, although long-term follow-up data are not yet available. Its use should be confined to tertiary referral centers.

When there is concomitant aortic stenosis, it is customary to deal with the most severe lesion first. A joint surgical and catheter laboratory-based approach may be optimal.

Repair of aortic aneurysm has until now involved major vascular surgical repair. The use of covered wall stents in selected patients may be a less traumatic option but again requires expertise in a tertiary center.

Medical management

Primarily, this is management of the associated complications of hypertension, left ventricular hypertrophy and accelerated atherosclerotic disease. ACE inhibitors and beta-blockers are particularly effective, although ACE inhibitors should be avoided in those with significant repair site gradients or in women considering pregnancy. Aggressive primary prevention for these patients is paramount and, therefore, should not be forgotten.

Examination

• Resting right arm blood pressure
• Nature and volume of femoral pulses
• Arm–leg blood pressure gradient (especially helpful)
• Resting saturations—normal
• Rhythm—usually sinus
• Heart sounds—systolic apical click from bicuspid aortic valve
• Murmurs—of repair site, collaterals, aortic valve disease including aortic regurgitation

Required follow-up

Coarctation patients need periodic follow-up at a specialist clinic. Those with known re-stenosis, small aneurysms and bicuspid aortic valve disease need close review. It is advisable that all patients have a baseline cardiac MRI (Fig. 12.2), which needs to be repeated periodically in those with any evidence of aneurysm formation. Cardiac MRA (angiography) has almost replaced invasive catheter investigations with regard to assessing re-coarctation and aneurysm formation (Fig. 12.3).

Pregnancy

Pregnancy carries a morbidity and mortality risk. Patients with unrepaired tight coarctation are at risk of severe hypertension, heart failure, stroke and aortic dissection. In addition, placental and fetal perfusion in such patients will be greatly diminished. In patients with repaired coarctation the risks are less, although there needs to be meticulous control of blood pressure, while avoiding placental and fetal hypoperfusion and drug-induced teratogenicity. Patients with aortic aneurysms and/or re-coarctation present a particular challenge. Pregnancy is contraindicated in those with a known significant aortic aneurysm. (See Chapter 3 for further details.)

Long-term outcome

• Outcome overall is good, although function may not return to normal even with early repair.

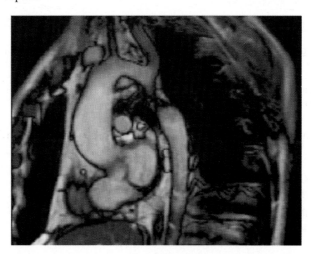

Fig. 12.2 Native coarctation of the aorta (cardiac MRI). Note marked dilatation of the left subclavian artery, proximal to coarctation suggesting excessive collateral flow. Also moderate ascending aortic dilatation, secondary to a coexistent bicuspid aortic valve. Ascending aortopathy is uncommon in patients with isolated aortic coarctation (without aortic valve involvement). Patient referred for primary stent implantation (transcatheter intervention).

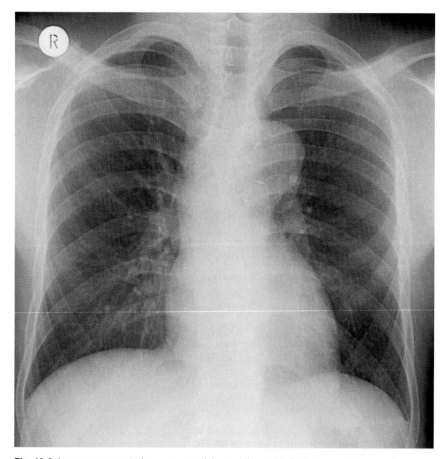

Fig. 12.3 Large paracoarctation aneurysm (chest radiograph). Patient presenting with hemoptysis and systemic hypertension many years after previous surgical repair of coarctation (note surgical clips) and referred for emergency surgery. Smaller aortic aneurysms may not be seen with chest radiography and we recommend routine cardiac MRI for all patients with previous repair of aortic coarctation.

• The commonest cause of death is atherosclerotic disease. Meticulous blood pressure control and addressing other risk factors may impact on prognosis. There may be justification for treating coarctation patients as secondary prevention subjects.

Endocarditis recommendations
For life! For all patients with coarctation (treated or untreated).

Exercise
Patients with repaired coarctation should be encouraged to exercise regularly. However, extreme isometric exercise should be avoided, especially by hypertensive patients.

Complications

- Arrhythmia: rare.
- Endocarditis: often difficult to detect; need low index of suspicion.
- Systemic hypertension: common.
- Ventricular dysfunction: rare unless hypertensive heart disease or aortic valve disease.
- Thrombotic events: rare.
- Sudden death: rare unless ruptured aortic or berry aneurysm.

Lesion-specific complications
- Repair site aneurysm, especially patch grafts (no longer used routinely).
- Re-coarctation: common.
- Accelerated atherosclerosis.
- Stroke disease: hemorrhagic and ischemic (including berry aneurysms).
- Ascending aortopathy.
- Aortic valve disease: stenosis or regurgitation.

Key clinical points

- Hemoptysis requires urgent aortic imaging with CT or MRI and referral to a tertiary center as it may herald aortic dissection or ruptured aneurysm.
- Low index of suspicion for ischemic heart disease.
- Meticulous control of blood pressure, lifelong.
- Coexisting re-coarctation may be missed in the setting of aortic valve disease—need a low index of suspicion.
- Pregnancy may present significant problems for these patients and should not be undertaken without specialist advice.

Further reading

Bromberg BI, Beekman RH, Rocchini AP, et al. (1989) Aortic aneurysm after patch aortoplasty repair of coarctation: a prospective analysis of prevalence, screening tests and risks. Journal of the American College of Cardiology, **14**(3), 734–741.

de Divitiis M, Pilla C, Kattenhorn M, et al. (2001) Vascular dysfunction after repair of coarctation of the aorta: impact of early surgery. Circulation, **104**(12), I165–70.

Hornung TS, Benson LN & McLaughlin PR (2002) Catheter interventions in adult patients with congenital heart disease. Current Cardiology Reports, **4**(1), 54–62.

Swan L, Wilson N, Houston AB, et al. (1998) The long-term management of the patient with an aortic coarctation repair. European Heart Journal, **19**(3), 382–386.

Toro-Salazar OH, Steinberger J, Thomas W, et al. (2002) Long-term follow-up of patients after coarctation of the aorta repair. American Journal of Cardiology, **89**(5), 541–547.

CHAPTER 13

Complete Transposition of the Great Arteries

Description of the lesion

In patients with complete transposition of the great arteries (TGA; Fig. 13.1), there is atrioventricular concordance and ventriculoarterial discordance—i.e. the right atrium connects to the morphological right ventricle which gives rise to the aorta and the left atrium connects to the morphologic left ventricle which gives rise to the pulmonary artery (Fig. 13.2). Consequently, the pulmonary and systemic circulations are connected in parallel rather than the normal in-series connection. This situation is incompatible with life unless mixing of the two circuits occurs.

Presentation and course in childhood

Newborns are typically pink at birth but become progressively cyanotic as the ductus closes. Survival before surgical repair is dependent upon mixing of the circulations at one level or another, whether natural (ventricular septal defect, VSD; atrial septal defect, ASD; patent ductus arteriosus, PDA) or by intervention (Blalock-Hanlon atrial septectomy or Rashkind balloon atrial septostomy).

Unoperated transposition is a lethal condition with 90% mortality by the age of one year. Nearly all patients will have had surgical intervention (atrial switch (Fig. 13.3), arterial switch, or Rastelli operation—see below) early on, with the exception perhaps of patients with a large VSD who may survive into

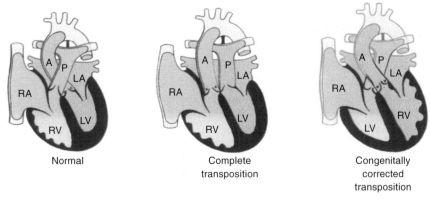

Normal   Complete   Congenitally
                      transposition   corrected
                                              transposition

Fig.13.1 Transposition of great arteries. Left panel: normal heart. Middle panel: complete (or simple) transposition—patients present with cyanosis soon after birth. Right panel: congenitally corrected transposition—patients present usually later depending on associated lesions (see Chapter 14). RA, right atrium; RV, right ventricle; LA, left atrium; LV, left ventricle; P, pulmonary trunk; A, aorta.

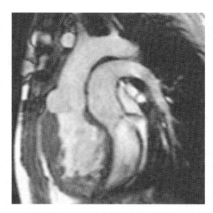

Fig. 13.2 Complete transposition of great arteries (cardiac MRI). Note anterior aorta arising from a hypertrophied systemic right ventricle (left part) and posterior pulmonary artery arising from the left ventricle. Note banana-shaped left ventricle (right lower panel) due to right ventricular dilatation. Patients with transposition complexes have a systemic right ventricle. The latter—despite adaptation and remodeling to support the systemic load—is associated with late ventricular dysfunction and failure in a proportion of patients.

adulthood without intervention and present with pulmonary vascular disease.

Physical examination

- *Atrial switch*: right ventricular parasternal lift, a normal S_1, a single loud S_2 (P_2 is not heard because of its posterior location), a holosystolic murmur from tricuspid regurgitation if present.
- *Arterial switch*: appears normal on physical examination. Diastolic murmur from neo-aortic valve regurgitation and systolic ejection murmur from right ventricular outflow tract obstruction (RVOTO) may be present.

Useful investigations

- **EKG**: sinus bradycardia or junctional rhythm, in the absence of a right atrial overload pattern, with evidence of right ventricular hypertrophy is characteristically present in patients following the *atrial switch* procedure. The EKG is typically normal in patients following the *arterial switch* procedure.
- **Chest radiography**: on the posteroanterior film, a narrow vascular pedicle with an oblong cardiac silhouette ('egg on its side') is typically seen in patients following the *atrial switch* procedure. For the *arterial switch*, normal mediastinal borders.
- **Echocardiography**: following the *atrial switch* procedure, parallel great arteries are the hallmark of TGA. Qualitative assessment of systemic right ventricular function, the degree of tricuspid regurgitation and the presence or absence of subpulmonic left ventricular obstruction (dynamic or fixed) is possible. Assessment of baffle leak or obstruction is best done using color and Doppler flow.

After *arterial switch*, neo-aortic valve regurgitation, supravalvar pulmonary stenosis and segmental wall motion abnormality from ischemia due to coronary ostial stenosis should be sought. In patients with the *Rastelli operation*, left ventricular to aorta tunnel obstruction as well as right ventricular to pulmonary artery conduit degeneration (stenosis/regurgitation) must be sought.

Surgical management

• *Atrial switch* (see Figs 13.2 and 13.3) (Mustard or Senning procedure): blood is redirected at the atrial level using a baffle made of Dacron® or pericardium (Mustard operation) or atrial flaps (Senning operation), achieving physiologic correction. Systemic venous return is diverted through the mitral valve into the subpulmonary morphologic left ventricle and the pulmonary venous return is rerouted via the tricuspid valve into the subaortic morphologic right ventricle. By virtue of this repair, the morphologic right ventricle is left to support the systemic circulation.

• *Arterial switch* (Jatene procedure): blood is redirected at the great artery level by switching the aorta and pulmonary arteries such that the morphologic left ventricle becomes the subaortic ventricle and supports the systemic circulation, and the morphologic right ventricle becomes the subpulmonary ventricle.

• *Rastelli procedure* (for patients with VSD and pulmonary/subpulmonary stenosis): blood is redirected at the ventricular level with the left ventricle tunneled to the aorta via the VSD and a valved conduit placed from the right ven-

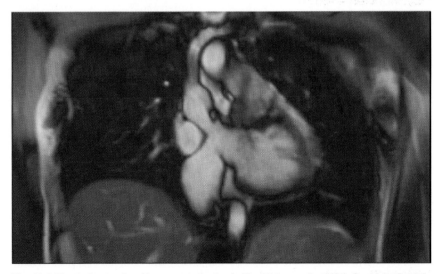

Fig. 13.3 Mustard procedure (the same patient as in Fig. 13.2—cardiac MRI). Consists of atrial redirection of flow to correct cyanosis. Patient continues to have the right ventricle supporting the systemic circulation. Mild stenosis of the superior vena cava part of the baffle (anastomosis) is seen at the left upper panel, leading to dilatation of the inferior vena cava anastomosis at the left bottom panel. Some of the drainage of the upper systemic venous blood is facilitated via the azygous system (not seen in this figure). Systemic veins drain into the smooth trabeculated left ventricle at the right bottom part of figure.

tricle to the pulmonary artery. By virtue of this procedure, the left ventricle supports the systemic circulation.

Late complications
- Following *atrial switch* procedure, one of the following complications may occur:
  - significant systemic (tricuspid) atrioventricular (AV) valve regurgitation (40%);
  - systemic right ventricular dysfunction (40%);
  - symptomatic bradycardia (sinus node dysfunction, AV node block) (50%)
  - atrial flutter and fibrillation (20% by age 20);
  - superior or inferior vena cava pathway obstruction;
  - pulmonary venous obstruction (rare);
  - atrial baffle leak.
- Following *arterial switch* procedure, the following complications may occur:
  - right ventricular outflow tract obstruction;
  - neo-aortic valve regurgitation;
  - myocardial ischemia from coronary artery obstruction.
- Following the *Rastelli procedure*, the following complications may occur:
  - right ventricle-to-pulmonary artery conduit stenosis;
  - significant subaortic obstruction (across LV–aorta tunnel);
  - residual VSD.

Recommended follow-up
Regular follow-up by physicians with special expertise in adult congenital heart disease is recommended.
- *Atrial switch*: serial follow-up of systemic right ventricular function is warranted. Echocardiography and RNA can be used, although MRI is especially useful.
- *Arterial switch*: regular follow-up with echocardiography is recommended.
- *Rastelli*: regular follow-up with echocardiography is warranted given the inevitability of conduit degeneration over time.
- Holter monitoring is recommended to diagnose unacceptable brady- or tachyarrhythmias.

Endocarditis recommendations
- All patients with DTGA status after atrial switch or Rastelli procedure should take SBE prophylaxis for life.
- Patients with DTGA status after arterial switch should take SBE prophylaxis if any residual hemodynamic disturbances are present (mild pulmonary stenosis, aortic regurgitation, etc.).

Exercise
- In the absence of severe cardiomegaly or severe pulmonary hypertension, patients should be restricted to class 1A type activities (see Chapter 6).

• Patients with severe cardiomegaly or severe pulmonary hypertension should not exercise.

Pregnancy and contraception

Pregnancy in women with a normal functional class following *atrial* switch operation is usually well tolerated. Worsening of systemic right ventricular function during or shortly after pregnancy, however, has been reported. ACE inhibitors should be stopped before pregnancy occurs.

Long-term outcome

• Atrial switch
  – Following atrial baffle surgery, most patients reaching adulthood will be in NYHA class I–II.
  – Progressive systemic right ventricular dysfunction and left AV valve regurgitation is the rule.
  – About 10% of patients will present with frank symptoms of congestive heart failure.
  – Atrial flutter/fibrillation occurs in 20% of patients by age 20.
  – Progressive sinus node dysfunction is seen in half of the patients by early adulthood.
• Arterial switch
  – Supravalvar pulmonary stenosis.
  – Ostial coronary artery disease.
  – Progressive neo-aortic valve regurgitation.
• Rastelli procedure
  – Progressive right ventricular to pulmonary artery conduit obstruction can cause exercise intolerance or right ventricular angina.
  – Left ventricular tunnel obstruction can present as dyspnea or syncope.

Key clinical points

• Patients with an *atrial* switch procedure and severe systemic (tricuspid) AV valve regurgitation may need:
  – valve replacement if systemic ventricular function is adequate;
  – consideration of heart transplantation;
  – a conversion procedure to an *arterial* switch following retraining of the left ventricle with a pulmonary artery band.
• Following an atrial switch procedure, atrial tachyarrhythmias and/or bradycardia commonly develop in early adulthood.

Corrected Transposition of the Great Arteries

Description of the lesion

In congenitally corrected transposition of the great arteries (L-TGA or CCTGA), the connections of both the atria to ventricles and of the ventricles to the great arteries are discordant. Systemic venous blood passes from the right atrium through a mitral valve to the left ventricle and then to the right-sided posteriorly located pulmonary artery. Pulmonary venous blood passes from the left atrium through a tricuspid valve to the right ventricle and then to an anterior, left-sided aorta (see Fig. 13.1). The circulation is thus 'physiologically' corrected, but the morphologic right ventricle supports the systemic circulation.

Associated anomalies occur in up to 98% and include:

- VSD (~75%);
- pulmonary or subpulmonary stenosis (~75%);
- left-sided (tricuspid and often 'Ebstein-like') valve anomalies (>75%);
- complete AV block (~2% per year).

Incidence and etiology

Congenitally corrected transposition of the great arteries is a rare condition, accounting for less than 1% of all congenital heart disease.

Presentation and course in childhood

Patients with *no associated defects* (~1% of all such patients) are acyanotic and often asymptomatic until late adulthood. Dyspnea and exercise intolerance from systemic ventricular failure and significant left AV valve regurgitation will usually manifest itself by the fourth or fifth decade, and palpitations from supraventricular arrhythmias may arise in the fifth or sixth decade.

Patients with a VSD and pulmonary outflow tract obstruction will either present in congestive heart failure (if VSD large) or cyanosed (if RVOTO severe) and will undergo classic repair (VSD patch closure with RVOT relief of obstruction) or double switch operation (atrial and arterial switch procedure) early on.

Significant left AV valve regurgitation is rarely seen in childhood and is more likely to arise later on or after classic repair type surgery.

Physical examination

- A single loud S_2 (A_2) will be heard, P_2 being silent due to its posterior location. The murmur of an associated VSD or left atrioventricular valve regurgitation may be heard. The murmur of pulmonary stenosis will radiate upward and to the right, given the rightward direction of the main pulmonary artery.
- If complete heart block is present, cannon A waves with an S_1 of variable intensity will be present.

Useful investigations

- **EKG**: complete atrioventricular block can be present. The presence of Q wave in leads V_{1-2} combined with an absent Q wave in leads V_{5-6} is typical and reflects the initial right-to-left septal depolarization occurring in the setting of 'ventricular inversion'. This should not be mistaken for evidence of previous anterior myocardial infarction.
- **Chest radiography**: because of the unusual position of the great vessels (pulmonary artery to the right and aorta to the left), the pulmonary trunk is

inconspicuous and an abnormal bulge along the left side of the cardiac contour reflects the left-sided ascending aorta rising to the aortic knuckle.

Surgical management

• *Classic repair*: this procedure consists of VSD patch closure, left ventricular to pulmonary artery valved conduit insertion and systemic tricuspid valve replacement. Patients having undergone 'classic' repair continue to have a morphologic right ventricle supporting the systemic circulation.

• *Double switch operation*: This procedure consist of an atrial switch procedure (Mustard or Senning) together with an arterial switch procedure. It should be considered for patients with severe tricuspid regurgitation and systemic ventricular dysfunction. Its purpose is to relocate the left ventricle into the systemic circulation and the right ventricle into the pulmonary circulation, achieving 'anatomic' correction. Firstly, the LV must be appropriately 'trained'.

• Complete AV block may require *pacemaker implantation* for symptoms, progressive or profound bradycardia, poor exercise heart rate response or cardiac enlargement.

Late complications

Natural history after *'classic' repair*:
• progressive systemic (tricuspid) AV valve regurgitation;
• progressive systemic (right) ventricular dysfunction;
• atrial arrhythmias;
• *acquired* complete atrioventricular block continues to develop at 2% per year, and is especially common at the time of heart surgery (25%);
• subpulmonary (morphologic left) ventricular dysfunction.

Recommended follow-up

All patients should have at least annual cardiology follow-up with an expert in the care of adult patients with congenital cardiac defects. Regular assessment of systemic (tricuspid) atrioventricular valve regurgitation by serial echocardiographic studies and systemic ventricular function by MRI (preferably) should be performed. Holter recording may be useful if paroxysmal atrial arrhythmias or transient complete AV block is suspected.

Endocarditis recommendations

• Unoperated CCTGA with associated left atrioventricular valve regurgitation, subPS or VSD should observe endocarditis prophylaxis for life.
• Patients who have undergone classic repair with residual lesions, prosthetic LAVV or double switch should practice SBE prophylaxis for life.

Exercise

• In the absence of severe pulmonary hypertension or cardiomegaly, patients with CCTGA should restrict their activities to class 1A types.

• Patients with severe cardiomegaly or severe pulmonary hypertension should not exercise.

Pregnancy

Pregnancy may be associated with a marked deterioration in systemic right ventricular function and/or the development or worsening of systemic (tricuspid) AV valve regurgitation. Moderate to severe systemic ventricular dysfunction as well as the presence of cyanosis prepartum increases maternal morbidity and fetal losses. Close supervision of such pregnant patients is recommended.

Key clinical points

• Left AV valve replacement should be performed before systemic right ventricular function deteriorates, namely at an ejection fraction ≥45%.
• Left AV valve repair is usually unsuccessful because of the abnormal, often 'Ebstein-like', anatomy of the valve.

Further reading

Transposition of the great arteries

Chang AC, Wernovsky G, Wessel DL, *et al.* (1992) Surgical management of late right ventricular failure after Mustard or Senning repair. *Circulation,* **86,** 140–149.

Flinn CJ, Wolff GS, Dick M, *et al.* (1984) Cardiac rhythm after the Mustard operation for complete transposition of the great arteries. *New England Journal of Medicine,* **310,** 1635–1638.

Gelatt M, Hamilton RM, McBride BW, *et al.* (1997) Arrhythmia and mortality after the Mustard procedure: a 30-year single-centre experience. *Journal of the American College of Cardiology,* **29,** 194–201.

Gewillig M, Cullen S, Mertens B, Lesaffre E & Deanfield J (1991) Risk factors for arrhythmia and death after Mustard operation for simple transposition of the great arteries. *Circulation,* **84,** 187–192.

Helvind MH, McCarthy JF, Imamura M, *et al.* (1998) Ventricular-arterial discordance: switching the morphologically left ventricle into the systemic circulation after 3 months of age. *European Journal of Cardiothoracic Surgery,* **14,** 173–178.

Kanter J, Papagiannis J, Carboi MP, Ungerleider RM, Sanders WE & Wharton JM (2000) Radiofrequency catheter ablation of supraventricular tachycardia substrates after Mustard and Senning operations for d-transposition of the great arteries. *Journal of the American College of Cardiology,* **35,** 428–441.

Puley G, Siu S, Connelly M, *et al.* (1999) Arrhythmia and survival in patients >18 years of age after the Mustard procedure for complete transposition of the great arteries. *American Journal of Cardiology,* **83,** 1080–1084.

Wilson NJ, Clarkson PM, Barratt-Boyes BG, *et al.* (1998) Long-term outcome after the Mustard repair for simple transposition of the great arteries: 28-year follow-up. *Journal of the American College of Cardiology,* **32,** 758–765.

Congenitally corrected transposition of the great arteries

Connelly MS, Liu PP, Williams WG, Webb GD, Robertson P & McLaughlin PR (1996) Congenitally corrected transposition of the great arteries in the adult: functional status and complications [see comments]. *Journal of the American College of Cardiology*, **27**, 1238–1243.

Imai Y (1997) Double-switch operation for congenitally corrected transposition. *Advances in Cardiac Surgery*, **9**, 65–86.

Presbitero P, Somerville J, Rabajoli F, Stone S & Conte MR (1995) Corrected transposition of the great arteries without associated defects in adult patients: clinical profile and follow up. *British Heart Journal*, **74**, 57–59.

Prieto LR, Hordof AJ, Secic M, Rosenbaum MS & Gersony WM (1998) Progressive tricuspid valve disease in patients with congenitally corrected transposition of the great arteries. *Circulation*, **98**, 997–1005.

van Son JA, Danielson GK, Huhta JC, *et al.* (1995) Late results of systemic atrioventricular valve replacement in corrected transposition. *Journal of Thoracic and Cardiovascular Surgery*, **109**, 642–652; discussion 652–653.

Van Praagh R, Papagiannis J, Grunenfelder J, Bartram U & Martanovic P (1998) Pathologic anatomy of corrected transposition of the great arteries: medical and surgical implications. *American Heart Journal*, **135**, 772–785.

Voskuil M, Hazekamp MG, Kroft LJ, *et al.* (1999) Postsurgical course of patients with congenitally corrected transposition of the great arteries. *American Journal of Cardiology*, **83**, 558–562. ·

CHAPTER 14

The Single Ventricle and Fontan Circulations

Description of the lesion

The Fontan surgery is a palliative procedure for individuals in whom a two-ventricular repair is not feasible, such as in tricuspid atresia, pulmonary atresia with intact ventricular septum or various types of univentricular hearts. The univentricle heart is selected as the representative defect for further discussion (Fig. 14.1).

In this defect, usually both atrioventricular (AV) valves are connected to a single ventricular cavity (double-inlet ventricle). This main ventricle is connected to a rudimentary chamber through a bulboventricular foramen. One great artery arises from the ventricle and the other from the rudimentary chamber. The single ventricle is left-type in 80% of cases. Transposition of the great arteries occurs in 85% of cases with the most common form being 'double inlet left ventricle with L-TGA' (aorta arising from the rudimentary chamber). Pulmonary stenosis or atresia is present in about half the cases, providing some protection to the pulmonary vasculature. Those cases without obstruction to pulmonary blood flow have high flow to the lungs.

Associated lesions
These include coarctation of the aorta, interrupted aortic arch and patent ductus arteriosus.

Incidence and etiology

• Single ventricle accounts for less than 1% of congenital defects.
• The defects in the category of 'single ventricle physiology' comprise a small percentage of congenital defects, but are some of the most complex.

Presentation and course in childhood

Because systemic and pulmonary blood are mixed in one ventricle, cyanosis is present. The severity of cyanosis depends on pulmonary blood flow.
• If pulmonary blood flow is increased, cyanosis is mild and the presentation is similar to transposition of the great arteries (TGA) with ventricular septal defect (VSD). Signs and symptoms of congestive heart failure may be prominent.
• If pulmonary blood flow is reduced, cyanosis is more severe and the presentation is similar to tetralogy of Fallot.

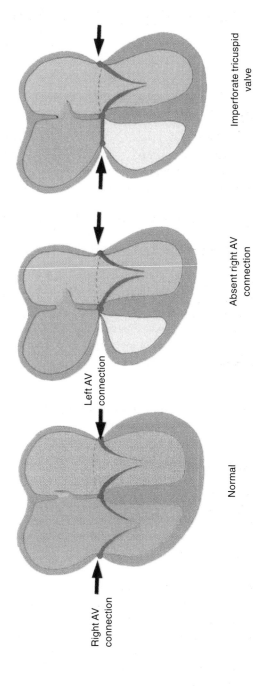

Fig. 14.1 'Single ventricle physiology'. Left panel: normal heart. Middle panel: patient with absent right AV connection (also called classical tricuspid atresia). Right panel: patient with imperforate tricuspid valve. 'Single ventricle' denotes a heart and a circulation which is not suitable for biventricular repair. Most patients with so-called 'single ventricle physiology' will be considered for a Fontan type of operation. Note the necessity of an adequate atrial septal defect, as there is no direct communication of the right atrium (and the systemic venous return) to the right ventricle. AV, atrioventricular.

Examination

- If pulmonary blood flow is increased:
  - mild cyanosis;
  - congestive heart failure/pneumonia;
  - 3–4/6 systolic ejection murmur at the left sternal border;
  - S_3;
  - apical diastolic rumble (high flow through the AV valves).
- If pulmonary blood flow is reduced:
  - moderate to severe cyanosis;
  - single S_2;
  - systolic ejection murmur at left sternal border (pulmonary stenosis).

Useful investigations

- **EKG**: unusual pattern of hypertrophy with similar appearing QRS complex across the precordium. First- or second-degree heart block may be present.
- **Chest radiography**: either increased or decreased pulmonary blood flow.
- **Echocardiography**:
  - two AV valves opening into a single ventricle;
  - rudimentary chamber;
  - bulboventricular foramen that may be obstructive;
  - transposition of the great arteries (D or L type);
  - obstruction of the pulmonary and/or aortic valve;
  - abnormalities of the AV valves;
  - associated defects.
- **MRI**:
  - is useful for assessment of anatomy and ventricular function (Fig. 14.2).

Catheter/surgical management

Palliative procedures include:
- a systemic to pulmonary artery (PA) shunt for severe cyanosis with associated pulmonary stenosis or pulmonary atresia;
- banding of the pulmonary artery if the bulboventricular foramen is not obstructive.

The Fontan surgery (Fig. 14.3) is the reparative surgery when a two-ventricle circulation is not possible. In this surgery, the systemic venous return is diverted to the pulmonary arteries, usually without passing through a subpulmonary ventricle. The current modification is the total cavo-pulmonary connection (TCPC) with or without a fenestration. This consists of the following.
- An end-to-side anastomosis of the superior vena cava (SVC) to the top of the right PA (bidirectional Glenn, Fig. 14.3); flow from the SVC is directed toward the right PA.

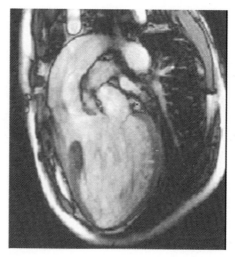

Fig. 14.2 'Single ventricle physiology' in a patient with double inlet left ventricle (cardiac MRI). Note anterior aorta (top left part of figure) arising from a rudimentary pouch-like anterior right ventricle. Main ventricle with smooth trabeculations dilated and posteriorly placed (right bottom part of figure) of left ventricular morphology. Smaller pulmonary trunk behind the aorta due to valvar and subvalvar pulmonary stenosis.

- An end-to-side anastomosis of the cardiac end of the SVC to the underside of the right PA, but offset slightly from the SVC to right PA anastomosis to direct flow toward the left PA.
- A tubular conduit from the orifice of the IVC to the orifice of the SVC. The conduit can be placed extracardiac (Fig. 14.3) or intracardiac (within the right atrium).

This can be performed as a single or two-stage procedure. If staged, a bidirectional Glenn anastomosis is performed first, followed by completion of the Fontan. The advantages of the Fontan procedure are normal or near-normal arterial oxygen content and removal of the volume overload of the single ventricle.

The following preoperative criteria identify individuals who do well after surgery.

- Mean pulmonary artery pressure ≤15 mmHg.
- Pulmonary vascular resistance ≤4 units/m^2.
- Ratio of pulmonary artery/aorta diameter ≥0.75 without distortion or narrowing of the pulmonary arteries.
- Systemic ventricular ejection fraction ≥60% and ventricular end-diastolic pressure ≤12 mmHg.
- Systemic valve regurgitation not greater than mild.

Individuals who meet these criteria have an 81% survival over 10 years. Survival falls to 60–70%, however, when one or more of these criteria are not met.

In individuals judged at higher surgical risk, a fenestration, 4–6 mm hole in the conduit is added. This prevents excessive elevations of right atrial pressure

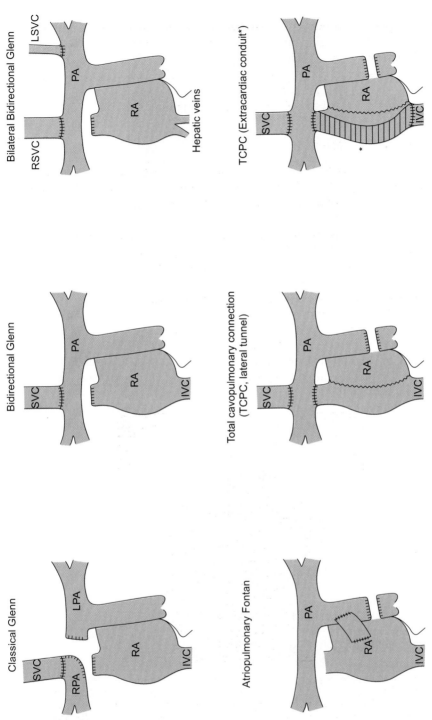

Fig. 14.3 Types of venous anastomoses and Fontan operations. See text. RPA, right pulmonary artery; SVC, superior vena cava; LPA, left pulmonary artery; RA, right atrium; IVC, inferior vena cava; PA, pulmonary artery; RSVC, right superior vena cava; LSVC, left superior vena cava; TCPC, total cavo-pulmonary connection; *, conduit or prosthetic tube.

and increases cardiac output in exchange for some hypoxemia. If the pressure in the Fontan circuit falls postoperatively, the fenestration can be closed with an atrial septal defect occlusion device.

Earlier versions of the Fontan procedure likely to be seen in adults include:
- direct right atrial appendage-to-pulmonary artery connection;
- formation of a lateral tunnel within the right atrium (Fig. 14.4).

Late complications

The complexity of congenital heart disease and the surgical procedure combined with the physiology of passive flow through the pulmonary circuit leads to an impressive list of complications. These include:
- arrhythmias, mostly supraventricular;
- intracardiac thrombus and thromboembolic events, either pulmonary or systemic (Fig. 14.5);
- severe right atrial enlargement (earlier Fontan version);
- protein-losing enteropathy;
- pulmonary vein obstruction due to right atrial enlargement;
- obstruction in the Fontan circuit;
- progressive systemic ventricular dysfunction and heart failure;
- progressive AV valve regurgitation;
- persistent right-sided pleural effusion;
- hepatic congestion and dysfunction;

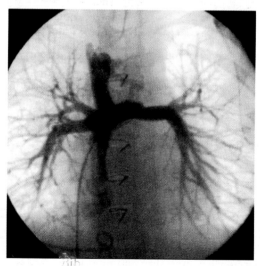

Fig. 14.4 Total cavopulmonary connection (TCPC) in a patient with tricuspid atresia (angiogram). Note direct anastomosis of the superior vena cava with the right pulmonary artery (top part of figure) and the catheter (bottom left part of figure) through the inferior vena cava and the intra-atrial baffle pointing to the lower end of the TCPC anastomosis. This operation is also called the lateral tunnel Fontan of TCPC.

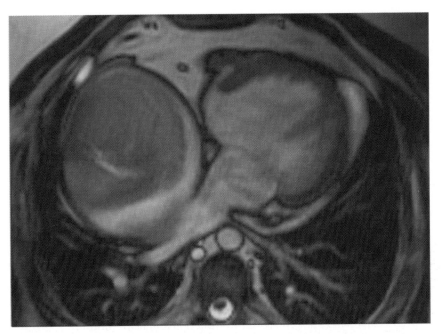

Fig. 14.5 Massive thrombus and marked right atrial dilatation in patient with a previous atrio-pulmonary Fontan operation (cardiac MRI). Thrombus occupies more than 80% of the massively dilated right atrium (left part of figure). Patient referred for conversion to an extracardiac type of total cavopulmonary connection (with thrombectomy, right atrial reduction and arrhythmia targeting surgery).

- cyanosis;
- pulmonary arteriovenous malformations or systemic-venous collaterals;
- sinus or AV node dysfunction with need for pacemaker placement;
- reoperation for revision or obstruction in the Fontan circuit or ventricular outflow tract obstruction.

Next, each of these complications is discussed and Table 14.1 summarizes their management.

Arrhythmia

Supraventricular tachycardia and bradyarrhythmias are common. Supraventricular tachyarrhythmias (atrial flutter or incisional atrial re-entrant tachycardia, atrial fibrillation, and atrial tachycardia) are common, occur with increasing frequency with longer follow-up, and often cause hemodynamic deterioration. About 5% of Fontan patients develop atrial arrhythmias per year, leading to important mortality and morbidity. Restoration and maintenance of sinus rhythm are, therefore, important.

Medical options for achieving this are cardioversion, catheter ablation procedures, pacing, or antiarrhythmic therapy (poor efficacy). A search for a hemodynamic problem as a precipitating factor is essential. Relieving such problems may eliminate or, more commonly, enable better control of the arrhythmia. Anticoagulation therapy is usually indicated once an arrhythmia occurs, as formation of atrial thrombus is more likely to develop. Conversion to a TCPC with concomitant MAZE type procedure may be considered.

Sinus and AV node dysfunction may require a pacemaker. Sinus node dysfunction with intact AV node is common and may just require transvenous atrial pacing. If AV node dysfunction is present, a dual-chamber pacemaker may need to be placed using epicardial leads. Medications that cause bradycardia or block at the AV node should be used with caution.

- *Types of arrhythmias*
  - Sinus node dysfunction with junctional rhythm (common).
  - AV node dysfunction.
  - Supraventricular tachyarrhythmias.
  - Atrial flutter, atypical (incisional atrial re-entrant tachycardia).
  - Atrial fibrillation.
  - Ventricular tachyarrhythmias.
- *Management of bradyarrhythmias*
  - Atrial pacing if AV node intact.
  - Dual-chamber pacing if AV node disease (epicardial leads).
- *Management of supraventricular tachyarrhythmias*
  - Restore sinus rhythm (pharmacological/cardioversion).
  - Maintain sinus rhythm.
- Antiarrhythmic therapy, improve hemodynamics, catheter ablation, surgery to revise Fontan plus arrhythmia surgery.
- Other issues
  - Anticoagulation for stroke risk reduction.

Thrombus/emboli

Sluggish, swirling blood flow in an enlarged right atrium with an atriopulmonary connection creates a high potential for thrombus. Atrial arrhythmias increase the risk of thrombus in all Fontan circuits, as does loss of proteins needed for coagulation (see protein-losing enteropathy). The incidence of thrombus is difficult to establish but is somewhere around 17–44%.

The management of thrombus and the use of anticoagulants in the Fontan are difficult issues. If an option, revision of the Fontan circuit with removal of the thrombus would be the recommendation of many. Indications for anticoagulants range from use in all individuals with a Fontan to selective use in those with tachyarrhythmias, a fenestration, enlarged right atrium with sluggish flow, or a clinical event consistent with embolus.

Ventricular dysfunction/heart failure

Although unproven, the usual therapy for left ventricle dysfunction is applied to this situation. However, caution is needed in the use of angiotensin-converting enzyme inhibitors as these may reduce preload.

Protein-losing enteropathy (PLE)

This is a serious complication with significant mortality and morbidity, which occurs in 4–13% of patients after a Fontan operation. Chronically increased systemic venous pressure and reduced cardiac output are associated with a severe loss of serum protein into the intestine. The consequences of the reduced serum oncotic pressure are generalized edema, ascites, pleural effusions and diarrhea (excessive intestinal protein loss and fat malabsorption).

Laboratory tests show low serum albumin and protein with low plasma but high stool levels of alpha-1-antitrypsin (A-1-AT). The 5-year survival after diagnosis is about 50%.

Diagnosis is established by documenting increased A-1-AT clearance with a 24-hour stool collection and a blood sample. Hypoalbuminemia and lymphopenia are associated abnormalities.

No treatment is universally effective, but the best success in treating PLE is to find a reversible cardiovascular abnormality. Therapies include high-protein diets, diuretics, steroids (prednisolone 1–2 mg/kg/day for 14–21 days), unfractionated heparin, somatostatin, 1–4 μg/kg twice or four times a day and therapy focusing on improving cardiac output (angiotensin-converting enzyme inhibitors and inotropic agents).

The interventional (catheter fenestration) and surgical repair of hemodynamic abnormality (revision of Fontan) should be considered early, before cachexia or chronic PLE are present. Heart transplantation is another option for refractory PLE.

Obstruction in the Fontan circuit

The development or worsening of symptoms or any of the complications listed in Table 14.1 should alert one to obstruction in the Fontan circuit and trigger a thorough investigation. Stenting or surgical revision is a consideration when obstruction is present.

Cyanosis/hypoxemia

Individuals without atrial fenestration usually have a transcutaneous oxygen saturation of ≥94%. An oxygen saturation below 90% may be due to:
- leakage across the inter-atrial baffle or previous fenestration site;
- venous collaterals draining into the left atrium;
- pulmonary AV malformations (classic Glenn procedure);
- alternatively, increased peripheral oxygen extraction from reduced cardiac output.

Collateral vessels may be coil embolized if needed. Pulmonary AV malformations may regress following reoperation to include the hepatic veins into the pulmonary circulation.

Hepatic dysfunction

Chronic mild hepatic congestion and mild hepatomegaly are typically due to

Table 14.1 Management of complications

Complication	Medical treatment	Catheter treatment	Surgical treatment
Atrial arrhythmias	Anti-arrhythmic therapy	Ablation	TCPC/MAZE
Thrombus in Fontan circuit	Anticoagulation therapy		TCPC
Obstruction in Fontan circuit		Dilatation/stent	Reoperation
Intra-atrial shunt/fenestration		Device closure	Reoperation
Pulmonary AV fistulas			Reoperation with inclusion of hepatic vein into the pulmonary circuit
Protein-losing enteropathy	Medication	Fenestration	Reoperation
Right pulmonary vein occlusion			TCPC
AV valve regurgitation	Afterload reduction		Repair/replacement
Ventricular outflow obstruction	Afterload reduction		Reoperation
Conduction abnormalities		Pacemaker (transvenous)	Pacemaker (epicardial)
Refractory heart failure			Heart transplantation

the high venous pressure in Fontan circuit and are usually not of clinical importance.

Surgical or catheter procedures to address these complications fall into five categories. Individuals may have a combination of procedures done.

1 Conversion of atriopulmonary connection to a total cavopulmonary connection (TCPC) for arrhythmias or poor hemodynamics associated with severe right atrial enlargement.

2 Correction of specific abnormality such as:

(a) systemic AV valve regurgitation not secondary to ventricular dysfunction;

(b) obstruction in the Fontan circuit (stenting or surgical);

(c) relief of ventricular outflow tract obstruction;

(d) replacement of dysfunctional conduit;

(e) fenestration in atrial septum for PLE (stenting or surgical);

(f) closure of fenestration or residual shunts (catheter or surgical).

3 Arrhythmia (ablation or surgical with right atrial maze or maze-Cox III cryoablation).

4 Pacemaker insertion (transvenous for sinus node disease or epicardial for AV node disease).

5 Heart transplantation.

Fontan patients with an atriopulmonary connection tend to have more complications than those repaired using total cavopulmonary connection (TPCP). Early data indicate considerable beneficial effects of TCPC conversion combined with arrhythmia surgery for Fontan patients with complications amenable to these procedures. This surgery is quite daunting. Long-term follow-up is needed to confirm persistence of benefits, and to determine if complications occur less frequently after conversion to TCPC.

Conduits need replacement for obstruction (kinking, hyperplasia of fibrous tissue, and thrombus). In the venous Fontan circuit, small pressure gradients of 2–4 mmHg can indicate significant obstruction.

Heart transplantation is an option in those with severe ventricular dysfunction unrelated to reversible anatomic problems or arrhythmias.

Required follow-up

These are some of the most complicated patients and require close follow-up in a congenital heart disease center to detect and promptly address any of the long list of complications that may occur.

Evaluation usually includes:

- history and clinical examination with transcutaneous oximetry;
- EKG to evaluate for arrhythmias or conduction abnormalities;
- chest radiography for cardiac size and status of pulmonary vasculature;
- blood tests for FFBC, electrolytes, serum protein and albumin levels;
- imaging studies to look for:
  - systemic ventricular function, AV valve regurgitation,

- thrombus/obstruction in the Fontan circuit,
- obstruction of right pulmonary veins,
- size of right atrium (atrio-pulmonary connection),
- right-to-left shunting.

Pregnancy and contraception

Many issues need to be considered in assessing the risks associated with becoming pregnant. Pregnancy may have significant risks due to the increased volume load on the single ventricle and further elevation of systemic venous pressure. This may cause symptoms of heart failure due to worsening ventricular function, AV valve regurgitation, or arrhythmias. The hypercoagulable state of pregnancy increases the concern for thrombus. The risk of spontaneous abortion is increased. Many women will be on medications that adversely affect the fetus. These include warfarin, angiotensin-converting enzyme inhibitors and amiodarone. The risk to the woman of stopping the medication needs to be weighed. While alternative medications are available, they may not be as effective as those replaced. However, with careful monitoring of cardiac and obstetric parameters, women with good exercise capacity, no history of tachyarrhythmias or previous embolic event and no significant hemodynamic concerns can undergo pregnancy successfully at relatively low risk.

Long-term outcome

The Fontan operation is palliative. The 10-year survival rate is 60–80%. Major causes of death include ventricular failure, arrhythmias, reoperation and PLE.

Endocarditis prophylaxis

Antibiotic prophylaxis is recommended in all patients.

Exercise

Individuals with the Fontan procedure have the most severe limitation of exercise capacity amongst patients with congenital heart disease. While their exercise capacity is reduced, they can exercise to their limits of comfort without significant risk. Competitive sports and extremes of exertion should be discouraged. Contact sports should be avoided for patients on warfarin.

Key clinical points

- The Fontan operation is a palliative, complicated surgery with unique physiology.
- The incidence of complications is high.
- Individuals with this complicated physiology should be followed every 6–12 months by an adult congenital heart disease cardiologist.

• Symptoms and arrhythmias require a thorough evaluation for underlying hemodynamic abnormalities.
• A combination of medical, interventional, and surgical procedures may be necessary to address these underlying hemodynamic abnormalities.

Further reading

Deal BJ, Mavroudis C, Backer CL, Johnsrude CL & Rocchini AP (1999) Impact of arrhythmia circuit cryoablation during Fontan conversion for refractory atrial arrhythmias. *American Journal of Cardiology*, **83**, 563–568.

Freedom RM, Hamilton R, Yoo SJ, *et al.* (2000) The Fontan procedure: analysis of cohorts and late complications. *Cardiology in the Young*, **10**, 307–331.

Mair DD, Puga F & Danielson GK (2001) The Fontan procedure for tricuspid atresia: early and late results of a 25 year experience with 216 patients. *Journal of the American College of Cardiology*, **37**, 933–939.

Marcelleti CF, Hanley FL, Mavroudis C, *et al.* (2000) Revision of previous Fontan connection to total extracardiac cavopulmonary anastomosis: a multicenter experience. *Journal of Thoracic and Cardiovascular Surgery*, **119**, 340–346.

Tetralogy of Fallot and Right Ventricular Outflow Tract Disorders

Description of the lesion

The defect is due to antero-cephalad deviation of the outlet septum resulting in four features (see Fig. 15.1):

- a nonrestrictive ventricular septal defect (VSD);
- an overriding aorta;
- right ventricular outflow tract obstruction (RVOTO) which may be infundibular, valvar or (usually) a combination of both, with or without supravalvar or branch pulmonary artery stenosis;
- consequent right ventricular hypertrophy.

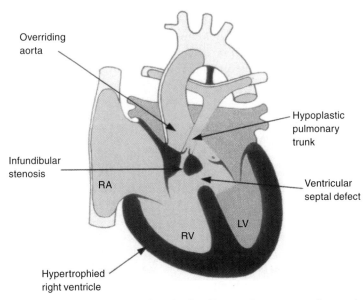

Fig. 15.1 Tetralogy of Fallot. Tetralogy (from the Greek) means four components, namely: infundibular stenosis (subvalvar pulmonary stenosis), ventricular septal defect, aortic overriding (of the ventricular septum) and secondary right ventricular hypertrophy. The pulmonary valve is usually dysplastic and stenotic too, and occasionally the pulmonary trunk (as per drawing) or distal pulmonary arteries can be hypoplastic or stenotic. RA, right atrium; RV, right ventricle; LV, left ventricle.

Incidence and etiology

• Tetralogy of Fallot is the most common form of cyanotic congenital heart disease after 1 year of age with an incidence approaching 10% of all forms of congenital heart disease.
• Approximately 15% of patients with tetralogy of Fallot have a deletion of chromosome 22q11.

Presentation and course in childhood

The clinical presentation varies depending on the degree of right ventricular outflow obstruction. With mild obstruction, the presentation is of increased pulmonary blood flow with dyspnea and minimal cyanosis, the so-called 'pink tetralogy' or 'acyanotic Fallot'. Most children, however, have significant RVOT obstruction with consequent right-to-left shunt and cyanosis.

Surgical management

• *Palliative procedures* (to increase pulmonary blood flow):
  – Blalock-Taussig shunt (classic or modified – subclavian artery to pulmonary artery end-to-side shunt or interposition graft);
  – Waterston shunt (ascending aorta to right pulmonary artery shunt);
  – Potts shunt (descending aorta to left pulmonary artery shunt).
• *Repair* (nowadays performed in infancy). Reparative surgery involves:
  – closing the ventricular septal defect with a Dacron® patch;
  – relieving the RVOT obstruction. The latter may involve resection of infundibular muscle, and insertion of a right ventricular outflow tract or transannular patch (Fig. 15.2).

Late complications

• *Palliation*: palliation was seldom intended as a permanent treatment strategy, and most of these patients should undergo surgical repair.
• *Repair*
  – *Pulmonary regurgitation*: significant pulmonary regurgitation (PR) is almost always encountered when the transannular patch repair technique has been employed. PR is usually well tolerated if mild to moderate. Severe chronic pulmonary regurgitation, however, may lead to symptomatic RV dilatation and dysfunction. The severity of pulmonary regurgitation, and its deleterious long-term effects, are augmented by coexisting proximal or distal pulmonary artery stenosis, or pulmonary artery hypertension (uncommon).
  – *Right ventricular (RV) dilatation*: RV dilatation is usually due to residual long-standing free PR +/– RVOT obstruction or as a consequence of RV surgical scar (transventricular approach for repair, now abandoned). Significant tricuspid

(a)
(b)

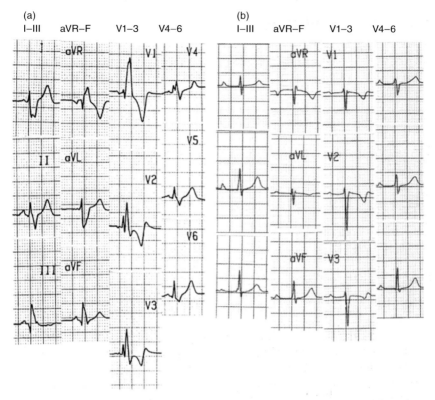

Fig. 15.2 Resting electrocardiogram from two patients with previous tetralogy repair. QRS duration after repair of tetralogy of Fallot relates to right ventricular size and the degree and rate of its prolongation—with time—predicts sustained ventricular tachycardia and sudden cardiac death. Left panel: patient with dilated right ventricle due to longstanding severe pulmonary regurgitation with a QRS duration of 180 ms. Patient presented with palpitations and shortness of breath and was referred for pulmonary valve implantation. Right panel: patient with mild residual pulmonary stenosis and no right ventricular dilatation. Note incomplete right bundle branch block pattern but narrow QRS complex. Low-risk subject for sustained ventricular tachycardia and sudden cardiac death.

regurgitation (TR) may occur as a consequence of RV dilatation, which begets more RV dilatation.

– *Residual right ventricular outflow tract (RVOT) obstruction*: residual RVOT obstruction can occur at the infundibulum, at the level of the pulmonary valve and main pulmonary trunk, distally, beyond the bifurcation and occasionally into the branches of the left and right pulmonary arteries (Fig. 15.3).

– *Aneurysmal dilatation of the RVOT*: this is relatively common in patients with previous transannular patch repair and significant pulmonary regurgitation. Aneurysmal dilatation of the RVOT can be associated with regional RV hypokinesis. Swirling of blood can be inferred from color flow Doppler signals in the aneurysmal right ventricular outflow tract regions. To date, no episodes of sudden rupture of these regions have been reported. Furthermore, this area can be the focus of sustained ventricular tachycardia.

– *Residual ventricular septal defect (VSD)*: residual VSDs can be encountered from either partial patch dehiscence or failure of complete closure at the time of surgery.

– *Aortic regurgitation (AR) with or without aortic root dilatation*: AR can be due to damage to the aortic valve during VSD closure or secondary to an intrinsic aortic root abnormality (more common in patients with pulmonary atresia and systemic to pulmonary artery collaterals). The pathologic substrate for aortic root dilatation seems to be 'cystic medial necrosis'.

– *Left ventricular dysfunction*: occasionally, left ventricular dysfunction can be seen from a variety of factors, including inadequate myocardial protection during previous repair(s), chronic LV volume overload due to longstanding palliative arterial shunts and/or residual VSD, injury to anomalous coronary artery (uncommon) or longstanding cyanosis before repair.

– *Endocarditis*: residual lesions leading to turbulent flow (residual VSD patch leak, RVOT obstruction, PR, TR) encountered in most patients after initial repair can serve as substrate for endocarditis.

– *Supraventricular arrhythmia*: atrial flutter and atrial fibrillation are relatively common in the current cohort of adults with previous tetralogy repair. Atrial tachyarrhythmia occurs in about one-third of adult patients and contributes to late morbidity and even mortality.

– *Ventricular tachycardia (VT)*: sustained monomorphic ventricular tachycardia is relatively uncommon. The usual arrhythmia focus is in the RVOT in the area of the previous infundibulectomy or VSD closure during tetralogy repair. Right ventricular dilatation from impaired hemodynamics is also contributory to the creation of re-entry circuits within the RV. The QRS duration from the standard surface EKG has been shown to correlate well with RV size in these patients (Fig. 15.2). A maximum QRS duration of 180 ms or more is a highly sensitive marker for sustained VT and sudden cardiac death in adult patients with previous repair of tetralogy.

– *Sudden cardiac death (SCD)*: the reported incidence of sudden death, presumably arrhythmic, in late follow-up series varies between 0.5–6% over 30 years, accounting for approximately one-third to one-half of late deaths.

Physical examination

• *Repaired*: parasternal right ventricular lift from right ventricular dilatation, a normal S_1 but a soft and delayed P_2 with a low-pitched diastolic murmur from pulmonary regurgitation at the left sternal border. A systolic ejection murmur from RVOTO, a high-pitched diastolic murmur from aortic regurgitation and a holosystolic murmur from a VSD patch leak can also be heard.

Useful investigations

• **EKG**: complete right bundle branch block following repair is the rule, especially if previous ventriculotomy. QRS width reflects the degree of right ventricular dilatation and is a prognostic marker for sustained ventricular tachycardia (VT) and sudden cardiac death (particularly when exceeds 180 ms).

• **Chest radiography**: following repair, cardiomegaly from right ventricular dilatation can be present. Dilatation of the ascending aorta can be seen.

• **Echocardiography**: following repair, residual pulmonary stenosis and regurgitation, residual VSD, right and left ventricular sizes and function, aortic root size, and the degree of aortic regurgitation should be assessed.

Recommended follow-up

All patients with tetralogy of Fallot (TOF), palliated or repaired, should have an annual cardiology follow-up. Particular attention should be paid to:

• degree of residual pulmonary regurgitation and or stenosis;

• degree of RV enlargement and RV systolic function (*preferably measured by MRI*) (Fig. 15.3);

• risk stratification: sustained VT and sudden cardiac death.

Endocarditis recommendations

All patients with repaired or unrepaired TOF should practice SBE prophylaxis for life.

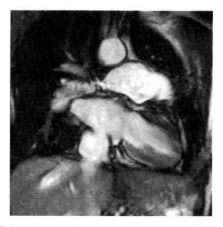

Fig. 15.3 Tetralogy of Fallot. Peripheral pulmonary artery stenosis after tetralogy repair (cardiac MRI). Patient with moderately severe origin stenosis of right pulmonary artery (RPA) seen at the top left panel with turbulent blood flow distally and severe pulmonary regurgitation (not seen here). Patient referred for transcatheter relief of RPA stenosis prior to surgical pulmonary valve implantation.

Exercise
• Patients without significant residual hemodynamic lesions, preserved bi-ventricular function, no aortic root dilatation and relatively short QRS duration need no exercise restriction.
• The remainder of clinically stable patients with repaired TOF should limit their activities to class 1A type.
• Patients with life-threatening arrhythmia should not exercise.

Pregnancy and contraception
• Pregnancy in unoperated patients constitutes a considerable risk of maternal and fetal complications and death. This risk is greater when resting oxygen saturations are <85%. The fall in peripheral resistance during pregnancy and hypotension during labor and delivery may increase the right-to-left shunt and aggravate pre-existing cyanosis.
• The risk of pregnancy in repaired patients depends largely on their hemodynamic status. The risk is low, approaching that of the general population, in patients with good underlying hemodynamics. In patients with significant residual RVOT obstruction, severe pulmonary regurgitation with or without tricuspid regurgitation and RV dysfunction, the increased volume load of pregnancy may lead to right heart failure and arrhythmias.
• All patients with tetralogy should have pre-conception cardiology counseling and follow-up by an adult congenital heart disease cardiologist during pregnancy. Pre-conception assessment of 22q11 deletion syndrome using fluorescent in situ hybridization (FISH) is recommended.

Long-term outcome

• The overall survival of patients who have had initial operative repair is excellent, with a 25-year survival of >94%.
• Over 85% of patients after intracardiac repair are asymptomatic on follow-up.
• Pulmonary valve replacement for chronic pulmonary regurgitation or RVOTO after initial intracardiac repair can be done safely with a mortality rate of 1%.
• Pulmonic valve replacement, when performed for significant pulmonary regurgitation, leads to an improvement in exercise tolerance as well as right ventricular dimension and function.
• Cryoablative procedures for VT combined with reoperations for hemodynamically significant lesions seem to lead to low recurrence rate of VT.

Key clinical points

• High-risk patients for sustained VT and/or sudden cardiac death include patients with right ventricular dilatation and a QRS duration ≥180 ms on their EKG.

- The development of major cardiac arrhythmias, most commonly atrial flutter/fibrillation or sustained ventricular tachycardia, usually reflects hemodynamic deterioration and should be treated accordingly with surgical repair of the hemodynamic disturbances as well as ablative intervention of the arrhythmia focus.
- Pulmonary valve replacement should be performed in patients with severe PR and RV dilatation.

Further reading

Gatzoulis MA, Till JA, Somerville J & Redington AN (1995) Mechanoelectrical interaction in tetralogy of Fallot. QRS prolongation relates to right ventricular size and predicts malignant ventricular arrhythmias and sudden death. *Circulation*, **92**, 231–237.

Gatzoulis MA, Balaji S, Webber SA, *et al.* (2000) Risk factors for arrhythmia and sudden death in repaired tetralogy of Fallot: a multi-centre study. *Lancet*, **356**, 975–981.

Ghai A, Silversides C, Harris L, Webb G, Siu Sam & Therrien J (2002) Left ventricular dysfunction is a risk factor for sudden cardiac death in adults late after repair of tetralogy of Fallot. *Journal of the American College of Cardiology*, **40**, 1675–1680.

Murphy JG, Gersh BJ, Mair DD, *et al.* (1993) Long-term outcome in patients undergoing surgical repair of tetralogy of Fallot [see comments]. *New England Journal of Medicine*, **329**, 593–599.

Nollert G, Fischlein T, Bouterwek S, *et al.* (1997) Long-term results of total repair of tetralogy of Fallot in adulthood: 35 years follow-up in 104 patients corrected at the age of 18 or older. *Thoracic and Cardiovascular Surgeon*, **45**, 178–181.

Nollert G, Fischlein T, Bouterwek S, Bohmer C, Klinner W & Reichart B (1997) Long-term survival in patients with repair of tetralogy of Fallot: 36-year follow-up of 490 survivors of the first year after surgical repair [see comments]. *Journal of the American College of Cardiology*, **30**, 1374–1383.

Therrien J, Siu S, Harris L, *et al.* (2001) Impact of pulmonary valve replacement on arrhythmia propensity late after repair of tetralogy of Fallot. *Circulation*, **103**, 2489–2494.

Therrien J, Marx GR & Gatzoulis MA (2002) Late problems in tetralogy of Fallot: recognition, management and prevention. *Cardiology Clinics*, **20**, 395–405.

Vliegen HW, van Strated A, de Roos A, *et al.* (2003) Magnetic resonance imaging to assess the hemodynamic effects of pulmonary valve replacement in adults late after repair of Tetralogy of Fallot. *Circulation*, **106**, 1703–1707.

CHAPTER 16

Pulmonary Atresia with Ventricular Septal Defect

Description of lesion

A percentage (~10%) of individuals with tetralogy of Fallot have pulmonary atresia rather than pulmonary stenosis. In addition to the unrestricted ventricular septal defect (VSD) and antero-cephalad deviation of the outlet septum, there is absence of direct communication between the right ventricular cavity and the pulmonary trunk. This lack of communication can be subvalvular/muscular (most common) or valvar. Another defining characteristic of this lesion is complex abnormalities of the pulmonary artery bed and its arterial supply. This lesion has also been referred to as 'pulmonary atresia with ventricular septal defect', but this is a broader term that also can include complete transposition of the great arteries, congenitally corrected transposition of the great arteries and double inlet ventricle. These lesions are distinct from 'tetralogy of Fallot with pulmonary atresia' and are not discussed in this chapter.

Pulmonary vascular anatomy and flow tends to have three patterns: one is described as unifocal circulation and two are multifocal (Fig. 16.1). In a unifocal circulation, all the intrapulmonary arteries are connected to unobstructed, confluent pulmonary arteries with blood supply from a patent duct (Fig. 16.1b). When different parts of a lung are supplied from more than one source, the circulation is described as multifocal. In one type, the branch pulmonary arteries are confluent but usually hypoplastic, since blood supply is from systemic to pulmonary artery collaterals (Fig. 16.1c). In the other multifocal pattern, blood flow also comes from multiple systemic to pulmonary arterial collaterals (MAPCAs), but the pulmonary arteries are non-confluent (Fig. 16.1d).

These arterial collateral vessels usually arise from the descending aorta opposite the origin of the intercostal arteries and extend to the origin of the intrapulmonary arteries at the segmental artery level near the hilum. In the multifocal patterns, total pulmonary vascular resistance (PVR) is difficult to quantitate when each pulmonary segment is supplied from a different arterial source. Pulmonary obstructive vascular disease may develop in a segment subjected to systemic pressure through a large nonrestrictive systemic-to-pulmonary artery collateral. Naturally occurring stenoses of such MAPCAs, however, may protect the lungs from systemic pressures and from the development of segmental pulmonary vascular disease. Sites of stenoses include:
- within the aorta to pulmonary collateral artery at its aortic end (most common)
- towards the pulmonary artery end
- at pulmonary arteriolar level.

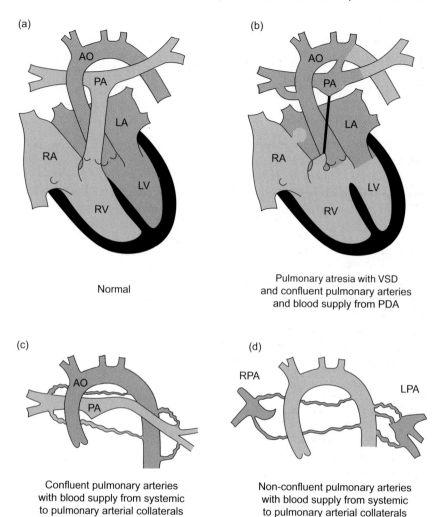

(a)

Normal

(b)

Pulmonary atresia with VSD
and confluent pulmonary arteries
and blood supply from PDA

(c)

Confluent pulmonary arteries
with blood supply from systemic
to pulmonary arterial collaterals

(d)

Non-confluent pulmonary arteries
with blood supply from systemic
to pulmonary arterial collaterals

Fig. 16.1 Three common patterns of pulmonary arterial anatomy in patients with tetralogy of Fallot with pulmonary atresia are shown. (b) Unifocal circulation with all the intrapulmonary arteries connected to unobstructed, confluent pulmonary arteries with blood supply from a patent duct. This is the most common pattern (85% of cases). (c) Multifocal circulation with confluent, but hypoplastic, pulmonary arteries and blood supply from systemic to pulmonary arterial collaterals. (d) Multifocal circulation with blood flow from systemic to pulmonary arterial collaterals, but the pulmonary arteries are non-confluent. AO, aorta; PA, pulmonary artery; RA, right atrium; LA, left atrium; RV, right ventricle; LV, left ventricle; RPA, right pulmonary artery; LPA, left pulmonary artery; VSD, ventricular septal defect; PDA, patent ductus arteriosus.

Incidence and etiology

Pulmonary atresia with ventricular septal defect (VSD) comprises about 1–2% of congenital heart defects. This lesion may be part of the 22q11 velo-cardiac syndrome (facial and aural anomalies, cleft palate, and developmental delay).

Presentation and course in childhood

Diagnosis is made in infancy with symptoms of cyanosis, failure to thrive and exertional dyspnea. Echocardiography, MRI and cardiac catheterization confirm the diagnosis. The overall prognosis is poor, but variable, depending upon the stability and adequacy of pulmonary blood flow. Prolonged survival without surgery is unlikely.

- If pulmonary flow is duct-dependent, cyanosis and symptoms worsen as the duct closes. Prostaglandin E1 infusion keeps the duct open until cardiac catheterization and surgery can be performed.
- Those with adequate, but not excessive, pulmonary blood flow can survive into adulthood without surgery. This well-balanced circulation occurs infrequently.
- Most commonly, individuals are stable, but lack adequate pulmonary blood flow. Long-term survival is guarded unless surgical intervention to improve pulmonary blood flow takes place.

Examination

- *Unrepaired patients*
  - Cyanosis.
  - No murmur or a continuous murmur from a patent ductus or systemic collateral flow to the lungs.
  - Single S_2.
- *Repaired patients*
  - With a valved conduit, a pulmonic ejection systolic with or without a regurgitant murmur.
  - Signs of right heart failure suggesting conduit or pulmonary artery obstruction.
  - Aortic regurgitation (secondary to aortic root dilatation).

Useful investigations

- **EKG**: EKG showing RAD and RVH.
- **Chest radiography**: boot-shaped cardiac silhouette and usually decreased pulmonary vascularity.
- **Echocardiography**: similar to tetralogy of Fallot plus absence of direct flow between the right ventricle (RV) and pulmonary artery (PA). Determine conduit function (in repaired patients), RV function, aortic root dilatation and the presence of aortic regurgitation.
- **Cardiac catheterization or MRI or CT**: to determine, size and confluence of pulmonary arteries, sources of pulmonary blood flow and pulmonary vascular resistance.

Surgical management

Individuals with palliative procedures or unoperated patients can be managed conservatively, if stable. If symptoms warrant, reparative surgery may be considered if irreversible pulmonary arterial obstructive disease is not present and the pulmonary anatomy is favorable.

The goals of reparative surgery are to close the VSD and to reconstruct the RV outflow tract and pulmonary vasculature. How this is achieved depends on the anatomy.

• The goal is easily achieved when pulmonary artery size is adequate (≥50% of normal) and the architecture is preserved (unifocalized circulation). The surgical approach is closure of the VSD and establishing continuity of the RV to the PA by a patch reconstruction or a valved conduit (homograft or heterograft tissue valve).

• When there are collaterals or hypoplastic pulmonary arteries, a single stage repair is not possible. One or more palliative surgical procedures are performed to promote growth of the pulmonary vasculature. Three options are possible.

– A systemic to pulmonary artery shunt (like a BT shunt).

– Right ventricular outflow tract reconstruction leaving the VSD open or at least fenestrated. This provides for more uniform enlargement of the pulmonary arteries.

– A central ascending aorta to pulmonary artery shunt. This must be the correct size to promote growth, without subjecting the lungs to excessive pulmonary blood flow.

Once pulmonary vasculature size has increased and pulmonary blood flow is adequate, complete repair may be considered. This includes closure of the VSD, and reconstruction of the RV outflow tract. Complete repair may not be advised if the PVR and RV systolic pressure remain significantly elevated.

• The most challenging group to repair has small, non-confluent pulmonary arteries (multifocal) with multiple collaterals supplying different regions of the lungs. A potential approach with this complex anatomy is to:

– maximize the number of lung segments perfused from a central pulmonary artery created by surgically connecting the collaterals together into a single source (unifocalization) of pulmonary blood flow, which in turn may or may not need insertion of a systemic to pulmonary shunt. This approach may require multiple surgeries;

– later attach these new branch pulmonary arteries to an RV to PA conduit, and close the VSD.

Catheter interventions include occluding, dilating, and stenting of branch pulmonary arteries and collateral arteries. Balloon valvuloplasty for stenosis of the conduit or valve is generally ineffective.

About 25–50% of patients are suitable and undergo this reparative approach. The remainder of patients either need no intervention or a small proportion may be suitable and are considered for heart–lung transplantation, although the results of the latter have been generally poor.

Reoperation

The long-term sequelae vary depending on the type of surgical palliation or repair. The need for reoperation is about 10–15% over 20 years. Replacement of the pulmonary conduit is a recurring issue (freedom from reoperation at 10 years is about 55% and at 20 years is 32%). Reoperation may be necessary for the following.
- *Revision of the RV outflow tract*
  - Residual infundibular stenosis: additional resection or placement of a new RV-to-PA conduit when RV systolic pressures is >75% of systemic pressure, especially with RV dysfunction.
  - Replacement of pulmonary valve in a conduit due to obstruction or regurgitation with progressive right heart enlargement.
  - Less commonly, an aneurysm of the RV outflow tract may develop and require resection.
- *Aortic valve replacement* for aortic regurgitation: progressive aortic regurgitation occurs more frequently in tetralogy of Fallot with pulmonary atresia than with tetralogy of Fallot with pulmonary stenosis.
- *Tricuspid valve repair* for significant regurgitation with progressive right heart enlargement. This is usually seen in association with significant RV outflow obstruction or insufficiency.
- *Residual VSD* if causing associated left heart volume overload.
- *Refractory atrial arrhythmias* may require radiofrequency surgical ablation or a Maze procedure. This is rarely done as the primary reason for surgery, but is added when surgery is needed for other indications.

Late complications

Causes of death in this population are mostly cardiac and include:
- cardiac surgery (43%);
- arrhythmias;
- non-cardiac surgery;
- chronic heart failure (excessive pulmonary blood flow, increased PVR, RV dysfunction, aortic regurgitation);
- hemoptysis;
- sudden death;
- endocarditis;
- increasing cyanosis (decreased pulmonary blood flow from collateral stenosis, PA stenosis, or increased PVR).

It is important to appreciate that while cardiac surgery enables these individuals to survive and improves cyanosis, it is also a major cause of mortality.

Despite the additional complexity of the abnormal pulmonary blood supply, the survival of repaired individuals may be similar to tetralogy of Fallot when hemodynamics are favorable (VSD is closed, right ventricular outflow tract obstruction is relieved, and pulmonary vascular resistance is at or near normal).

Survival falls to much lower levels, the more complex the pulmonary malformations and the less satisfactory the repair (survival in palliated patients of 61% at 20 years follow-up). Heart–lung transplantation may be an option when other options fail, but this is technically very difficult if extensive collateral vessels are present.

Follow-up

Patients with tetralogy of Fallot and pulmonary atresia should be followed up regularly by a cardiologist familiar with congenital heart disease in the adult. Symptoms such as dyspnea, increasing cyanosis, change in the shunt murmur, heart failure or arrhythmias warrant special attention.

Endocarditis prophylaxis
Endocarditis prophylaxis is recommended for all patients for life.

Exercise
Those with excellent hemodynamics will still have some reduced exercise capacity. They are, however, capable of meeting most physical demands. Those with less optimal hemodynamics will be more physically limited. Extremes of exertion or competitive contact are to be discouraged for the latter.

Pregnancy
The risk of pregnancy in repaired patients with good hemodynamics and no arrhythmias is low. The risk increases with hypoxemia (oxygen saturation <85%), pulmonary hypertension, ventricular dysfunction, heart failure symptoms and arrhythmias. DiGeorge status should be checked routinely prior to pregnancy.

Key clinical points

- Although pulmonary atresia with VSD shares many features with tetralogy of Fallot, the complex abnormalities of the pulmonary arteries and blood flow make it a much more challenging lesion to manage.
- Survival is poor without surgical intervention.
- Surgical management is quite diverse, depending on the complexity of the pulmonary circulation. It may be as simple as an RV-to-PA conduit, or it may require several procedures to connect multiple PA segments into a single source artery (unifocalization) before an RV-to-PA conduit can be performed.
- RV-to-PA conduits eventually need replacement.
- Mortality and morbidity are related to the
  - anatomic complexities;
  - completeness of the repair;
  - right ventricular function.

Further reading

Bull K, Somerville J, Ty E & Spiegelhalter D (1995) Presentation and attrition in complex pulmonary atresia. *Journal of the American College of Cardiology*, **25**, 491–499.

Cho JM, Puga FJ, Danielson GK, *et al.* (2002) Early and long-term results of the surgical treatment of tetralogy of Fallot with pulmonary atresia, with or without major aortopulmonary collateral arteries. *Journal of Thoracic and Cardiovascular Surgery*, **124**, 70–81.

Clarke DR & Bishop DA (1995) Ten year experience with pulmonary allografts in children. *Journal of Heart Valve Disease*, **4**, 384–391.

Dearani JA, Danielson GK, Puga FJ, *et al.* (2003) Late follow-up of 1095 patients undergoing operation for complex congenital heart disease utilizing pulmonary ventricle to pulmonary artery conduits. *Annals of Thoracic Surgery*, **74**, 399–411.

Leonard H, Derrick G, O'Sullivan J & Wren C (2000) Natural and unnatural history of pulmonary atresia. *Heart*, **84**, 499–503.

Murthy KS, Rao SG, Naik SK, Coelho R, Krishnan US & Cherian KM (1999) Evolving surgical management for ventricular septal defect, pulmonary atresia, and major aortopulmonary collateral arteries. *Annals of Thoracic Surgery*, **67**, 760–764.

Reddy VM, McElhinney DB, Amin Z, *et al.* (2000) Early and intermediate outcomes after repair of pulmonary atresia with ventricular septal defect and major aortopulmonary arterial collateral arteries. *Circulation*, **101**, 126–137.

CHAPTER 17

Ebstein's Anomaly of the Tricuspid Valve

Description of the lesion

Ebstein anomaly encompasses a wide spectrum of anatomic and functional abnormalities of the morphologic tricuspid valve (TV) that have certain features in common (see Fig. 17.1).

- Apical displacement of the septal and postero-lateral leaflets of the tricuspid valve below the atrioventricular junction into the right ventricle.
- Resultant 'atrialization' of the inflow of the right ventricle to varying degrees and consequently a smaller 'functional' right ventricle.
- Varying degrees of tricuspid regurgitation (occasionally, the tricuspid valve is stenotic).
- Enlargement of the right atrium.
- A shunt at atrial level, either patent foramen ovale (PFO) or secundum atrial septal defect (ASD), in approximately 50%.
- One or more accessory conduction pathways, increasing the risk of atrial tachycardias, in 25% of cases.

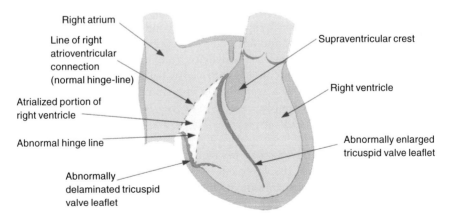

Fig.17.1 Ebstein anomaly of the tricuspid valve. Note the atrialized portion of the right ventricle (small in this case) caused by the displacement of the tricuspid valve towards the right ventricular apex.

Presentation and course in childhood

The presentation and natural history of patients with Ebstein anomaly depends on its severity. The fetus with extreme Ebstein anomaly will die in utero from hydrops fetalis. Children with severe Ebstein anomaly will present in infancy with failure to thrive and symptoms of congestive heart failure. Moderate Ebstein anomaly will manifest itself in adolescence with dyspnea and/or palpitations. Adults with Ebstein anomaly can remain asymptomatic throughout their life, or develop exercise intolerance, palpitations, cyanosis or paradoxical emboli from a right-to-left shunt at atrial level.

Physical examination

- Unimpressive jugular venous pressure because of the large and compliant right atrium and atrialized right ventricle.
- Widely split S_1 with a loud tricuspid component (the 'sail sound').
- Widely split S_2 from the right bundle branch block.
- Right-sided third heart sound.
- A holosystolic murmur increasing on inspiration from tricuspid regurgitation will be best heard at the lower left sternal border.
- Cyanosis from a right-to-left shunt at atrial level may or may not be present.

Useful investigations

- **EKG**: the EKG presentation of Ebstein anomaly varies widely (Fig. 17.2). Low voltage is typical. Peaked P waves in lead II and V_1 reflect right atrial enlargement. The PR interval is usually prolonged, but a short PR interval and a delta wave from early activation through an accessory pathway can be present. An RsR pattern consistent with right ventricular conduction delay is typically seen in lead V_1. Atrial flutter and fibrillation are common in the adult patient.
- **Chest radiography**: a rightward convexity from an enlarged right atrium and atrialized right ventricle coupled with a leftward convexity from a dilated infundibulum give the heart a 'water bottle' appearance on chest radiography (Fig. 17.3). Cardiomegaly, highly variable in degree, is the rule. The aorta and the pulmonary trunk are inconspicuous. The pulmonary vasculature is usually normal to reduced.
- **Echocardiography**: the diagnosis of Ebstein anomaly can often be made by echocardiography. Apical displacement of the septal leaflet of the tricuspid valve by 8 mm/m^2 or more, combined with an elongated sail-like appearance of the anterior leaflet will confirm the diagnosis.

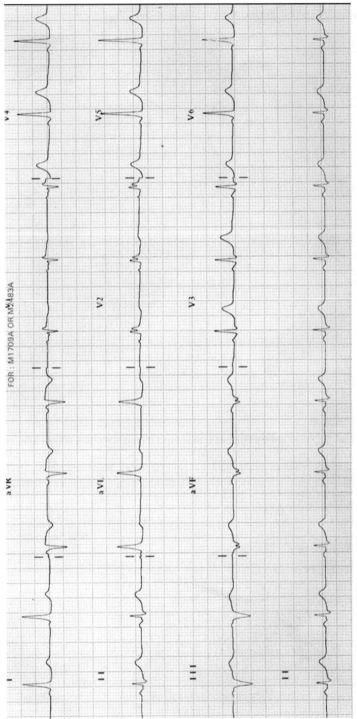

Fig. 17.2 Resting 12-lead electrocardiogram (EKG) from a patient with Ebstein anomaly of the tricuspid valve. Called the great mimic, EKG can vary from normal (rare) to grossly abnormal. Common features are low voltage QRS complexes, right bundle branch block pattern and/or left axis deviation (all present here) and abnormal P wave axis and configuration. Short PR interval and presence of delta waves (not present here) would suggest coexistence of Wolf-Parkinson-White syndrome.

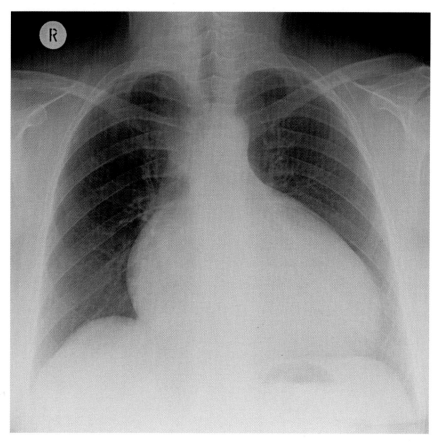

Fig. 17.3 Cardiomegaly in a patient with Ebstein anomaly of the tricuspid valve (chest radiograph). Cardiomegaly varies from minimal to extreme ('wall-to-wall' heart, presenting with either fetal death or severe neonatal cyanosis due to lung hypoplasia, secondary to a huge right atrium). Other typical features of isolated Ebstein anomaly are normal or reduced pulmonary vascular markings seen here, with a narrow pedicle (due to small pulmonary and aortic trunks, secondary to reduced cardiac output).

Surgical management

Indications for intervention include:
• deteriorating functional capacity (NYHA ≥ class III);
• progressive cyanosis;
• right-sided heart failure;
• occurrence of paradoxical emboli;
• recurrent supraventricular arrhythmias not controlled by medical or ablation therapy;
• asymptomatic progressive cardiomegaly (cardiothoracic ratio >65%).
  Surgery may involve the following:
• Tricuspid valve repair.

- If the tricuspid valve is not reparable, valve replacement will be necessary.
- The atrialized portion of the right ventricle is sometimes plicated at the time of surgery to reduce the risk of atrial arrhythmias.
- For 'high risk' patients, a bidirectional cavo-pulmonary connection may be added to reduce right ventricular preload (bidirectional Glenn).
- If present, cryoablation of the accessory pathway can be carried out at the time of surgery.
- Closure of PFO/ASD, if present.

Late complications

- Reoperation on a repaired tricuspid valve may be necessary if significant residual tricuspid regurgitation persist.
- Valve re-replacement may be necessary because of a failing bioprosthesis or thrombosed mechanical valve.
- Late arrhythmias can occur.
- Complete heart block after tricuspid valve replacement can occur.

Recommended follow-up

All patients with Ebstein anomaly should have regular follow-up, the frequency dictated by the severity of their disease. Particular attention should be paid to patients with:
- cyanosis;
- progressive asymptomatic cardiomegaly;
- worsening right ventricular function;
- recurrent atrial arrhythmias;
- progressive tricuspid regurgitation and/or stenosis following tricuspid valve repair/replacement.

Endocarditis recommendations
- All patients with repaired or unrepaired Ebstein anomaly should practice subacute bacterial endocarditis prophylaxis for life.

Exercise
- In the absence of severe cardiomegaly, all clinically stable Ebstein patients should limit their activities to class 1A type.
- In the presence of severe cardiomegaly or class IV symptoms, exercise is contraindicated.

Pregnancy
In the absence of maternal cyanosis, right-sided heart failure or arrhythmias, pregnancy is usually well tolerated.

Long-term outcome

With satisfactory valve repair, the medium-term prognosis is excellent. With valve replacement, results may be less satisfactory.

Key clinical points

- The diagnosis of Ebstein anomaly can normally be made by echocardiography. Apical displacement of the septal leaflet of the tricuspid valve by 8 mm/m^2 or more confirms the diagnosis.
- Progressive asymptomatic cardiomegaly is a relative indication for surgical repair.
- Tricuspid valve repair is preferable to replacement when feasible.

Further reading

Celermajer DS, Bull C, Till JA, *et al.* (1994) Ebstein's anomaly: presentation and outcome from fetus to adult. *Journal of the American College of Cardiology*, **23**, 170–176.

Chauvaud S, Fuzellier JF, Berrebi A, *et al.* (1998) Bi-directional cavopulmonary shunt associated with ventriculo and valvuloplasty in Ebstein's anomaly: benefits in high risk patients. *European Journal of Cardiothoracic Surgery*, **13**, 514–519.

Danielson GK, Driscoll DJ, Mair DD, Warnes CA & Oliver WC, Jr (1992) Operative treatment of Ebstein's anomaly. *Journal of Thoracic and Cardiovascular Surgery*, **104**, 1195–1202.

Shiina A, Seward JB, Edwards WD, Hagler DJ & Tajik AJ (1984) Two-dimensional echocardiographic spectrum of Ebstein's anomaly: detailed anatomic assessment. *Journal of the American College of Cardiology*, **3**, 356–370.

Shiina A, Seward JB, Tajik AJ, Hagler DJ & Danielson GK (1983) Two-dimensional echocardiographic–surgical correlation in Ebstein's anomaly: preoperative determination of patients requiring tricuspid valve plication vs replacement. *Circulation*, **68**, 534–544.

CHAPTER 18

Patent Arterial Duct

Description of the lesion

Patent arterial duct or patent ductus arteriosus (PDA) is a vessel communication connecting the proximal left pulmonary artery to the descending aorta just distal to the left subclavian artery (Fig. 18.1). During fetal life, PDA is a vital structure bypassing the pulmonary circulation by diverting blood flow from the right ventricle to the descending aorta. PDA was first described by Galen in AD 131.

The size and shape of the patent arterial duct vary greatly and impact on pathophysiology and on the type of occluding device when catheter intervention is considered.

From the clinical perspective, PDA during adulthood can be graded as follows.

- *Silent*: tiny PDA detected only by non-clinical means (usually echocardiography); no heart murmurs audible.

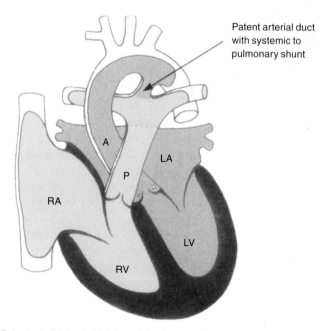

Fig. 18.1 Patent arterial duct with left-to-right shunting. RA, right atrium; RV, right ventricle; LA, left atrium; LV, left ventricle; A, aorta; P, pulmonary artery.

• *Small*: audible long-ejection or continuous murmur, radiating to the back. Causes negligible hemodynamic change. Normal peripheral pulses, normal left atrial and left ventricular size without any pulmonary hypertension.
• *Moderate*: wide, bouncy peripheral pulses (as with important aortic regurgitation). Audible, continuous murmur. Causes enlargement of the left atrium and left ventricle and some degree of pulmonary hypertension (usually reversible).
• *Large:* usually in adults with Eisenmenger physiology. Signs of pulmonary hypertension. Continuous murmur is absent. Causes differential cyanosis (lower body saturations lower than right arm saturations) and toe clubbing.

Associated lesions
• Associated lesions are common in pediatric patients.
• Coarctation of the aorta and a ventricular septal defect (VSD) are most common among them.
• Vascular ring (usually in the setting of a left-sided PDA with right aortic arch).
• PDA is universally present at birth in patients with congenital heart disease associated with limited or interrupted pulmonary or systemic blood flow (such as in patients with pulmonary atresia or the hypoplastic left heart syndrome, respectively). The circulation under these circumstances is PDA-dependent, and patency of the PDA is critical to survival until surgery is performed.

Incidence and etiology
• 12%; the third most common of congenital heart lesions.
• A common lesion in premature infants (0.8%) and with maternal rubella.

Presentation and course in childhood
• Most children with a PDA are asymptomatic.
• Neonates may present with heart failure when a large PDA is present, leading to excessive pulmonary blood flow (usually after the first week of life when pulmonary vascular resistance falls to lower, normal levels).
• Other infants may present with a heart murmur and bouncy pulses.
• Older children with a large, nonrestrictive PDA often develop irreversible pulmonary vascular disease (usually by the age of 18 to 24 months), which in turn down regulates pulmonary blood flow. Under these circumstances, a loud pulmonary component to the second heart sound is the more prominent feature with marked reduction or disappearance of the systolic heart murmur.

Course in adulthood
• Patients with *small, silent PDAs* have a normal life expectancy.
• Life expectancy is also normal in *patients who underwent surgical or catheter closure* of a PDA in infancy or early childhood. Attention should be paid to

patients who had some elevation of pulmonary vascular resistance at the time of PDA closure. Such patients may present later on in life with symptomatic pulmonary hypertension.

• Patients with *moderate size PDAs* may also present during adulthood (Fig. 18.2). Late presentation may be with a continuous murmur and bouncy pulses, or with the development of left heart dilatation and left-to-right shunt-related pulmonary hypertension. The majority of adult patients with a moderate PDA will ultimately become symptomatic with dyspnea and/or palpitations (atrial fibrillation, secondary to longstanding left atrial dilation), although frank heart failure may also occur.

• A *large PDA* is rare in the adult, most having been repaired in infancy and childhood. Pulmonary hypertension is usual and may not reverse entirely with closure of the defect. Many patients with a large PDA are symptomatic from dyspnea or palpitations. Eisenmenger PDA has a similar prognosis to Eisenmenger VSD, although symptoms may be less marked and exercise tolerance better (see Chapter 20).

Examination

• Oxygen saturations: should be normal with a small/moderate PDA. Differential cyanosis is present with a large PDA in the presence of pulmonary hypertension with lower body (post-PDA) desaturation patient with blue and clubbed feet and pink hands.

• Nature and volume of the femoral pulses.

• Bouncy or collapsing pulses: suggest significant aortic runoff with a large left-to-right shunt.

• Rhythm: usually sinus.

• Cardiac impulses: may be displaced to the left with large shunts and left heart dilatation.

• Continuous machinery murmur: common with moderate PDAs and left-to-right shunting, without pulmonary hypertension.

• Long, ejection systolic heart murmur: suggestive of a smaller PDA.

• Right ventricular lift: with pulmonary hypertension, secondary to a large, unrestrictive PDA.

• Diastolic heart murmur: mitral flow murmur at the apex.

• Pansystolic heart murmur: due to a small VSD.

Useful investigations

• **Chest radiography**: often normal; may show cardiomegaly (moderate to large PDA); PDA calcification may be present.

• **EKG**: usually normal; LVH with large PDA; RVH with pulmonary hypertension.

• **Echocardiography**: usually diagnostic (Fig. 18.2); transesophageal echocardiogram rarely indicated.

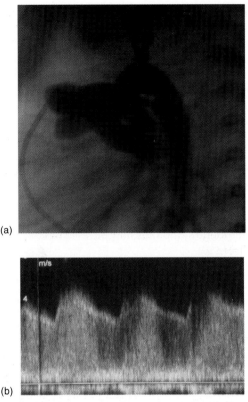

(a)

(b)

Fig. 18.2 Moderate patent arterial duct (angiogram and echocardiogram). (a) Aortic angiogram in patient with a small to moderate size 'restrictive' PDA prior to catheter closure. Restrictive denotes absence of irreversible pulmonary vascular disease. (b) Continuous wave Doppler from the same patient showing a high velocity exceeding 4 m/s during both systole and diastole, suggesting low pulmonary arterial pressures. Main indications for closure here are to reverse mild left heart dilatation due to volume overload and to eliminate the risk of endarteritis (low).

- **Cardiac catheter** (Fig. 18.2): for catheter device closure. Consider performing coronary angiography in patients older than 40 years of age.
- Other tests: not indicated.

PDA closure in adults should be considered in the following situations.
- The presence of a PDA, with the exception of (1) the silent tiny duct and (2) the presence of severe, irreversible pulmonary vascular disease.
- The occurrence of an episode of endarteritis, irrespective of the size of the PDA.
- *Closure of the tiny PDA, not audible on auscultation, remains controversial and should not be routinely performed,* despite the ease of transcatheter intervention, given the extremely low risk of endarteritis.
- If pulmonary hypertension is present (pulmonary arterial pressure >2/3 of systemic arterial pressure or pulmonary arteriolar resistance exceeding 2/3

of systemic arteriolar resistance), *there must be a net left-to-right shunt of 1.5:1 or more, or evidence of pulmonary artery reactivity* with reversibility studies *or, in highly selected cases, lung biopsy evidence that pulmonary arterial changes are potentially reversible.*

Catheter and surgical management

• Device closure is the preferred method for the majority of PDAs in most centers today. When possible, it should be planned at the same time as the 'diagnostic' cardiac catheterization. Pre-intervention transthoracic echocardiography usually provides indirect information on the magnitude of left-to-right shunt and on pulmonary arterial pressure.
• The presence of ductal calcification increases surgical risks and favors device closure. If surgical closure is pursued, for whatever reasons, such patients need ductal division, often under cardiopulmonary bypass, as PDA ligation alone is usually ineffective.
• Surgical closure should be reserved for patients with PDAs too large for device closure. Very occasionally, ductal anatomy may be so distorted (ductal aneurysm or post-endarteritis) as to make device closure undesirable.

Medical management

• This primarily is the management of the associated complications of left heart volume overload, atrial tachyarrhythmia and occasionally pulmonary hypertension (see Chapter 20 for management of patients with Eisenmenger physiology) when present.

Late outcomes

Catheter closure
• Successful closure (see Fig. 18.3) is achieved in the large majority of cases using a variety of devices.
• More than 85% of ducts are closed completely by 1 year following device implantation.
• Embolization of the device—usually in the left pulmonary artery—can occur but is uncommon, and usually the device can be retrieved percutaneously.
• In a small proportion of patients, a second or even a third device may need to be placed for complete closure. This is usually deferred for at least 6 months to a year from the first intervention, because of the potential for spontaneous closure.
• Recanalization is rare but can occur.

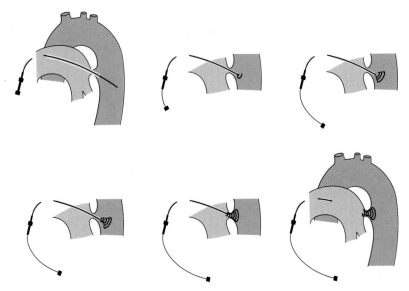

Fig. 18.3 Coil catheter closure of a small patent ductus arteriosus (PDA). Transvenous approach. Note delivery system via the pulmonary artery, through the PDA into the descending aorta (top left panel), distal part of the coil being released into the aorta (top middle and right panel), coil and the delivery system pulled back into the PDA ambula (bottom left and middle panel) and ultimately proximal part of the coil released and deployed with the delivery system being removed (bottom middle and right panel).

Surgical closure
• More than 95% of ducts can be closed by surgery. Recanalization is unusual but recognized.
• Postoperative complications may include recurrent laryngeal or phrenic nerve injury and thoracic duct damage.

Required follow-up

• Patients who have had surgical closure of a PDA may benefit from infrequent periodic evaluation by a cardiologist, because recanalization can occur, or residual problems (pulmonary hypertension, left ventricular dysfunction, atrial fibrillation) may persist or develop.
• Patients with devices in situ should also be considered for follow-up, as the long-term outcome of device closure remains unknown.

Endocarditis recommendations
• Endocarditis prophylaxis is recommended for 6 months following PDA device or surgical closure, or for life if any residual defect persists.
• Patients with a silent native PDA do not require follow-up or endocarditis prophylaxis.

Exercise
• Patients with a PDA and left-to-right shunt, in general, do not require any exercise restrictions.
• For those with pulmonary hypertension see Chapter 22 and the Eisenmenger complex see Chapter 20.

Pregnancy
Pregnancy is well tolerated in women with a PDA and left-to-right shunts.
• Congestive heart failure can occur in patients with moderate shunts and left heart dilatation at preconception. Such patients warrant cardiologic and specialist obstetric input during pregnancy and the peripartum.
• Patients with a clinically evident PDA should be considered for endocarditis prophylaxis at the time of delivery.
• Pregnancy is contraindicated in patients with a large PDA and Eisenmenger syndrome because of the high maternal and fetal mortality.

Late complications

• Endarteritis: rare.
• PDA aneurysm: common in young infants or after endarteritis; otherwise rare.
• PDA calcification: common in elderly patients.
• Atrial arrhythmia: late complication, with moderate PDAs.
• Ventricular dysfunction: late complication (as above).
• Progressive pulmonary hypertension: depends on the size of the PDA and the degree of left-to-right shunting. Occurs early—within the first 1 to 2 years of life—leading to irreversible pulmonary vascular disease in patients with very large PDAs and no restriction of flow. With time, patients develop Eisenmenger physiology, with differential cyanosis (to the lower body).

Key clinical points

• Large PDAs need early closure to prevent pulmonary hypertension.
• Moderate PDAs with left heart dilatation should also be closed electively for prognostic reasons (see text).
• Small, clinically silent ducts need no intervention or specific precautions.
• Catheter closure is the treatment of choice for the majority of PDAs in adulthood.
• Excellent prospects with normal survival for patients with closed PDAs and no residual pulmonary hypertension.
• Follow-up is required for patients with residual PDA communications (and endocarditis prophylaxis) and for patients with pulmonary hypertension.

Further reading

Campbell M (1968) Natural history of persistent ductus arteriosus. *British Heart Journal,* **30,** 4.

Cheung Y, Leung MP & Chau K (2001) Transcatheter closure of persistent arterial ducts with different types of coils. *American Heart Journal,* **141**(1), 87–91.

Faella HJ & Hijazi ZM (2000) Closure of the patent ductus arteriosus with the Amplatzer PDA device: immediate results of the international clinical trial. *Catheterization and Cardiovascular Interventions,* **51**(1), 50–54.

Mavroudis C, Backer CL & Gevitz M (1994) Forty-six years of patent ductus arteriosus division at Children's Memorial Hospital of Chicago. Standards for comparison. *Annals of Surgery,* **220**(3), 402–409.

Therrien J, Connelly MS & Webb GD (1999) Patent ductus arteriosus. *Current Treatment Options in Cardiovascular Medicine,* **4,** 341–346.

CHAPTER 19

Marfan Syndrome

Incidence and etiology

Marfan syndrome is a genetic condition manifesting an abnormality of elastin. It is inherited as an autosomal dominant trait, but penetrance is variable. The pathologic abnormality involves fragmentation of the medial elastic tissue in the aorta. The combination of a high amount of abnormal elastic tissue in the ascending aorta and the repetitive stress of ejection of blood probably leads to the gradual, but progressive aortic dilatation.

The estimated prevalence is 1 in 10,000 individuals. Spontaneous mutations occur in 20–30% of cases.

Fibrillin 1 is the primary glycoprotein component of elastin. Defects of this fibrillin gene on chromosome 15 are associated with Marfan syndrome. The defects, however, are usually unique in each family or sporadic case. More than 200 mutations have been identified so far, making the use of genetic markers for diagnosis unfeasible. Further confusion results as a mutation is not always found in those diagnosed with Marfan syndrome, while one may be found in individuals who do not meet the diagnostic criteria for Marfan syndrome.

Description of the lesion

While aortic root dilatation and dissection of the ascending aorta are the most defining abnormalities, other cardiac manifestations include mitral valve prolapse, calcification of the mitral annulus and dilatation of the main pulmonary artery. While mitral valve prolapse is common (70–90% of individuals), serious mitral regurgitation is relatively uncommon.

Associated lesions in the ocular and skeletal systems are essential in establishing the diagnosis of Marfan syndrome. Ectopia lentes (lens dislocation), myopia and retinal detachment (infrequent) are evident at an early age and tend to remain stable.

The musculoskeletal abnormalities tend to be the most obvious, often initiating the concern for Marfan syndrome. Common observations are dolichostenomelia (long, thin arms and legs), arachnodactyly (long, thin fingers), decreased ratio of upper body segment to lower segment, arm span greater than height, positive wrist and thumb sign, scoliosis, chest wall deformities (pectus excavatum or carinatum), and lax joints.

Other less specific manifestations include striae distensae (stretch marks) typically pectoral, deltoid, back, or thigh areas, spontaneous pneumothorax (11%) and dural ectasia (widening of the lumbosacral spinal canal).

As no specific laboratory or diagnostic test can establish the diagnosis of Marfan syndrome, major and minor criteria have been developed with the latest revision in 1996 (Ghent diagnostic criteria, Table 19.1). The major criteria are extremely uncommon in those without Marfan syndrome, while the minor criteria are frequently noted in the general population.

The diagnosis of Marfan syndrome de novo requires two major criteria in different organ systems and involvement of a third organ system. Only one major criteria plus involvement of a second organ system is necessary if the individual has a family history of the disease (parent, sibling, or child who meets diagnostic criteria independently).

Presentation and course in childhood

The diagnosis of Marfan syndrome can be made before adulthood in most

Table 19.1 Ghent diagnostic criteria

System	Major	Minor
Cardiovascular	Aortic root dilatation Dissection of ascending aorta	Mitral valve prolapse Mitral annular calcification (<40 years) Dilated main pulmonary artery Dilatation/dissection of descending aorta
Ocular	Lens dislocation	(2 needed to achieve minor criteria) Flat cornea Myopia Elongated globe
Skeletal	(4 = major criteria) Pectus excavatum needing surgery Pectus carinatum Pes planus Wrist and thumb sign§ Scoliosis >28° or spondylolisthesis Arm span/height ratio >1.05 or upper to lower segment ratio <0.86* Protrusio acetabulae (radiography or MRI)** Elbow extension (<170°)	Moderate pectus excavatum High, narrowly arched palate Typical facies Joint hypermobility
Pulmonary	None	Spontaneous pneumothorax Apical bulla
Skin	None	Unexplained stretch marks (striae) Recurrent or incisional hernia
Central nervous system	Lumbosacral dural ectasia (CT or MRI)**	None

§Thumb and 5th finger overlap around the wrist or the entire thumb nail projects beyond the ulnar border of the hand.
*Lower segment is the distance from symphysis pubis to floor and upper segment calculated by subtracting this distance from the height.
**Should only be done when a positive finding would establish the diagnosis.

cases. Infants who manifest Marfan syndrome have more problems with mitral valve prolapse and regurgitation than with aortic root dilatation. The mitral valve annulus is large and may calcify. Presentation with significant regurgitation of the mitral or aortic valve (due to aortic root enlargement) is more common than with aortic dissection or rupture.

Course in adulthood

Most individuals with Marfan syndrome will be asymptomatic. However, sudden death may still occur. Death is most commonly due to cardiovascular events with aortic rupture or dissection the most feared complications. If death is not sudden, an intense sharp pain between the shoulders, in the anterior part of the chest, or in the neck is typical for aortic dissection. A picture of circulatory collapse (shock state) could indicate a contained aortic rupture. A less common and less life-threatening presentation is heart failure with the findings of significant aortic or mitral regurgitation.

Since the rate of aortic root enlargement varies widely and unpredictably, it is essential to regularly assess aortic root size. This is usually done annually or more frequently if a sudden change is seen, or the size of the root is approaching the point when elective replacement is recommended. This is most commonly done by transthoracic echo (Fig. 19.1), but transesophageal echo, MRI and CT are all acceptable. Individuals should also be monitored for development of significant insufficiency of the aortic or mitral valve.

Examination

- See diagnostic criteria, Table 19.1.
- Aortic root enlargement occurs without symptoms or physical findings.
- A clinical picture of circulatory collapse (shock state) may indicate a contained aortic rupture.
- Findings of aortic insufficiency (diastolic decrescendo murmur, widened pulse pressure and bounding pulses) or mitral regurgitation (holosystolic murmur).

Useful investigations

- Establishment of the diagnosis using the Ghent diagnostic criteria.
- **Chest radiography**: aortic root dilatation.
- **Echocardiography**: aortic root dilatation at the sinuses of Valsalva (Fig. 19.1) and associated cardiac defects.
- **CT or MRI**: determination the diameter of the entire aorta. Also assessment of dural ectasia.

For children, nomograms are available to relate aortic root size to body surface area. In adults, aortic root diameter and body surface area do not correlate

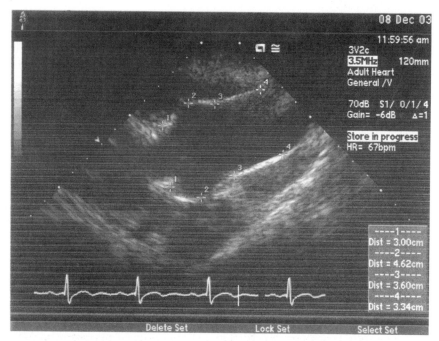

Fig. 19.1 A high parasternal long axis view of the aortic valve and ascending aorta in an individual with Marfan syndrome. Measurements should be made routinely in four positions: the annulus of the aortic valve (position 1), sinus of Valsalva (position 2), sinotabular junction (position 3) and ascending aorta (position 4). The enlargement of the aorta occurs most commonly at the sinus of Valsalva, as in this example showing a moderately enlarged aorta with a diameter of 46 mm.

well. One generally becomes concerned that the aortic root is dilated when it exceeds a diameter of 37 mm.

Surgical management

Table 19.2 summarizes surgical management of this condition. Urgent surgery is indicated for ascending aortic dissection and contained rupture. Aortic dissection arising beyond the left subclavian (not involving the ascending aorta) can be initially treated with medical therapy. Persistent symptoms or descending aortic diameter greater than 50 mm warrant surgical replacement.

While individuals with a normal or mildly dilated aortic root occasionally dissect, the risk of dissection increases as the aortic root enlarges. Elective replacement of the aorta should be considered when:
• the maximal diameter of the root exceeds 55 mm;
• the diameter exceeds 50 mm in an individual with a family history of aortic dissection/rupture or a rapidly change in size (>2 mm/year);
• the diameter exceeds 45 mm and pregnancy is desired or surgery is indicated for another reason (severe valvular regurgitation).

Table 19.2 Management based on diameter of aortic root

Aortic diameter (mm)	Management
<37	Normal limit for adults
≥37–44	Measure aortic root size yearly
≥45–49	1 Measure aortic root size yearly 2 Replace if • surgery for another cardiac indication • woman desiring pregnancy
≥50–54	1 Measure aortic root size every 6–12 months 2 Replace if • family history of dissection/rupture • rapid change in size (>2 mm/year)
≥55	Elective replacement (in all patients)

Replacement of the aorta with sparing of a normal aortic valve is potentially the ideal procedure. The modified Bentall is an alternative: replacement of the entire aortic root with a composite graft containing a mechanical, bioprosthetic or homograft valve. The distal end of the graft extends up to the brachiocephalic artery. The native coronary arteries are implanted into the graft. Some have questioned the long-term durability of the aortic valve in valve sparing operations. (See Fig. 19.2.)

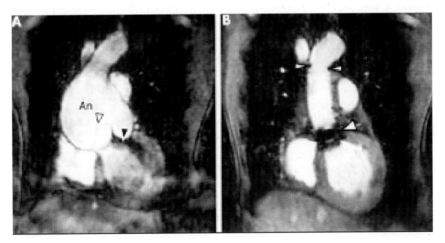

Fig. 19.2 Marked aortic root dilatation in a patient with Marfan syndrome before and after surgery (cardiac MRI). Left panel: patient with Marfan syndrome lost to follow-up presents with a large aortic root and ascending aortic aneurysm (An, maximum diameter 8.5 cm) with a dissection (white arrow) and aortic regurgitation. Right panel: same patient after emergency aortic root and valve replacement; arrows indicate the proximal and distal points of the anastomotic conduit. Preservation of the native aortic valve was not possible in this case, presenting late. With permission from Wong *et al.* (2002) *Heart,* **87**, 66.

Medical management

Beta-blockers are used to slow the progression of aortic dilatation and reduce the risk of dissection. They should be used in all Marfan patients at any age when aortic root diameter is ≥40 mm and even considered in those with a diameter <40 mm.

In those unable to tolerate beta-blockers, angiotensin-converting enzyme inhibitors (ACEi) or calcium antagonists are alternatives. If beta-blockers do not adequately control blood pressure, other antihypertensive medications should be added. While beta-blockers are beneficial, the individual should not feel that this is all that needs to be done. An important aspect of care is the regular assessment of the aortic diameter with elective intervention at the appropriate time.

Late complications

The reduced life expectancy in individuals with Marfan syndrome results from cardiovascular complications, with aortic rupture or dissection accounting for most deaths. Life expectancy in the 1970s averaged about 32 years of age. With regular follow-up evaluations, beta-blocker therapy and elective surgical treatment (aortic root replacement/aortic valve and root replacement), survival has improved significantly with average life expectancy about 60 years of age. The operative mortality for elective replacement is <2%, while it is 11.7% for emergency operations. Survival for elective replacement of the aortic root at 10 years is 75%. These results favor earlier elective intervention.

Required follow-up

Prior to surgery, yearly follow-up with assessment of aortic root size is recommended, with more frequent measures as the diameter approaches 50 mm. The risk for dissection and enlargement of the descending thoracic aortic is still present after replacement of the aortic root. Yearly follow-up with less frequent assessment of the aorta with MRI or CT is sufficient for most individuals.

Endocarditis prophylaxis

Endocarditis prophylaxis is recommended when there is mitral valve prolapse with regurgitation, after aortic valve replacement and after root replacement (6 months).

Exercise

Avoidance of contact sports and strenuous exertion and isometric exercise are recommended to reduce excessive stress on the proximal aorta.

Pregnancy

Pregnancy has two significant risks: one affects the child and the other involves the mother. Each offspring has a 50% chance of having Marfan syndrome. The mother risks progression of cardiovascular abnormalities, particularly aortic root dilatation, during pregnancy. Gestational hypertension and pre-eclampsia may increase this risk further. Beta-blockers should be continued throughout pregnancy. Pregnancy is considered relatively safe if the aortic diameter is less than 40 mm, a size at which dissection has rarely been reported. Conversely, at an aortic root diameter of 45 mm or greater, pregnancy is strongly discouraged. Elective surgery to replace the root should be considered prior to pregnancy. The risk of further dilatation or rupture when the aortic diameter is 40–45 mm is difficult to judge. In general, pregnancy is discouraged, more forcefully if aortic size has recently increased or the family history for aortic rupture/dissection is concerning, and less forcefully if these variables are absent.

Women with Marfan syndrome should have the aortic size carefully monitored during pregnancy, with the precise frequency determined by the assessed risk or concern for the individual.

Long-term outcome

Despite replacement of the aortic root, dissection and enlargement of the aortic arch or descending thoracic aortic is a lifelong risk. Although less common, hemodynamically significant aortic or mitral regurgitation can develop.

Key clinical points

- Mortality is primarily related to aortic root dissection or rupture, usually preceded by progressive aortic root enlargement.
- Progressive enlargement of the aorta is usually asymptomatic, therefore regular assessment of proximal aortic size is required.
- If aortic root enlargement is detected (>40 mm), beta-blocker therapy is indicated (perhaps for those under 40 mm too).
- Elective surgery to replace the dilated aorta when its diameter exceeds 55 mm, or 50 mm in high-risk patients.
- Elective surgery has very low mortality and dramatically improves survival.
- After surgical replacement of the aorta, individuals are still at risk for dissection or dilatation of the arch and descending thoracic aorta and need to be monitored yearly.

Further reading

Bassano C, De Matteis GM, Nardi P, *et al.* (2001) Mid-term follow-up of aortic root remodeling compared to Bentall operation. *European Journal of Cardiothoracic Surgery*, **19**, 601–605.
Dean JCS (2002) Management of Marfan syndrome. *Heart*, **88**, 97–103.

De Paepe A, Devereux RB, Dietz, *et al.* (1996) Revised diagnostic criteria for the Marfan syndrome. *American Journal of Medical Genetics*, **62**, 417–426.

Gott VL, Greene PS, Alejo DE, *et al.* (1999) Replacement of the aortic root in patients with Marfan syndrome. *New England Journal of Medicine*, **340**, 1307–1313.

Lind J & Wallenburg HCS (2001) The Marfan syndrome and pregnancy: a retrospective study in a Dutch population. *European Journal of Obstetrics Gynecology and Reproductive Biology*, **98**, 28–35.

Nollen GJ, Groenink M, van der Wall EE & Mulder BJM (2002) Current insights in diagnosis and management of the cardiovascular complications of Marfan syndrome. *Cardiology in the Young*, **12**, 320–327.

Roman MJ, Devereux RB, Kramer-Fox R, O'Loughlin J, Spitzer M & Robins J (1989) Two-dimensional echocardiographic aortic root dimensions in normal children and adults. *American Journal of Cardiology*, **64**, 507–512.

Rossiter JP, Repke JT, Morales AJ, Murphy EA & Pyeritz RE (1995) A prospective longitudinal evaluation of pregnancy in the Marfan syndrome. *American Journal of Obstetrics and Gynecology*, **173**, 1599–1606.

Shores J, Berger KR, Murphy EA & Pyeritz RE (1994) Progression of aortic dilatation and the benefit of long-term B-adrenergic blockade in Marfan syndrome. *New England Journal of Medicine*, **330**, 1335–1341.

CHAPTER 20

Eisenmenger Syndrome

Description of the lesion

Eisenmenger syndrome is pulmonary hypertension with a reversed central shunt. An uncorrected large central left-to-right shunt causes a progressive, eventually irreversible rise in pulmonary vascular resistance (PVR) leading to reversal of or bidirectional shunt flow with resultant hypoxemia. Pulmonary vascular obstructive disease induced by the high shunt flow is responsible for the progressive rise in PVR. While Dr Paul Wood identified 12 different congenital intracardiac or extracardiac defects that can cause Eisenmenger syndrome, ventricular septal defect (VSD) (Figs 20.1 and 20.2), atrioventricular (AV) septal defect and patent ductus arteriosus (PDA) account for 70–80% of cases. Less commonly seen defects are truncus arteriosus, surgically created aorto-pulmonary connections, complex pulmonary atresia and univentricular heart. With large shunts, the pulmonary vascular obstruction develops relatively quickly, usually within the first two years of life. An atrial septal defect (ASD) is associated with the Eisenmenger syndrome in adulthood, but it is debated whether this low-pressure shunt directly causes the irreversible pulmonary vascular obstructive disease, or whether it is due to recurrent pulmonary emboli or other secondary causes of pulmonary hypertension.

Associated lesions

No specific associated abnormalities are seen with the Eisenmenger syndrome. Associated lesions are related to the underlying congenital defect.

Incidence and etiology

Eisenmenger syndrome is not a congenital defect, but a pathophysiologic condition resulting from various arterial-to-venous shunt lesions. It is, fortunately, present in only a small number of patients followed in adult congenital heart disease programs.

Presentation and course in childhood

Children may be asymptomatic or have only mild symptoms of dyspnea. Reduced exercise capacity, dyspnea and fatigue develop gradually as pulmonary blood flow decreases, and hypoxemia increases due to bidirectional shunting. Despite cyanosis at rest and significantly impaired exercise capacity, most children with Eisenmenger syndrome do reasonably well. A slow, progressive decline occurs as they approach adulthood.

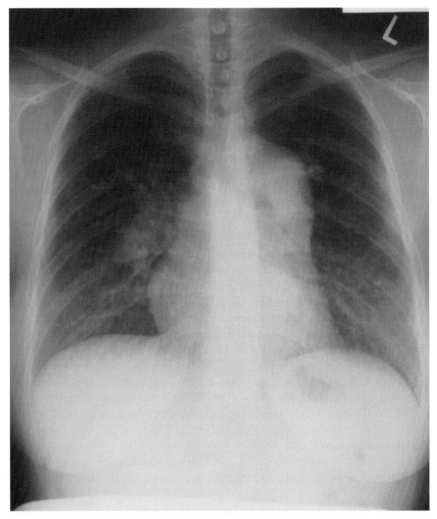

Fig. 20.1 Chest radiograph from a patient with Eisenmenger syndrome and a large VSD. Note mild cardiomegaly, marked right atrial dilatation and marked dilatation of central pulmonary arteries. Typical appearance of a young adult patient with compensated right ventricular hypertrophy and maintained right ventricular systolic function. Marked peripheral pulmonary artery 'prooning' not present (not a feaure of Eisenmenger physiology, in contrast to patients with primary acquired pulmonary arterial hypertension).

Course in adulthood

Many individuals with Eisenmenger syndrome survive into adulthood with 80% survival at 10 years, 77% survival at 15 years and 42% at 25 years after diagnosis. Variables associated with poor prognosis include syncope, elevated right atrial pressure and severe resting hypoxemia (<80% transcutaneous oxygen saturation). The attrition is progressive with causes of death listed below.

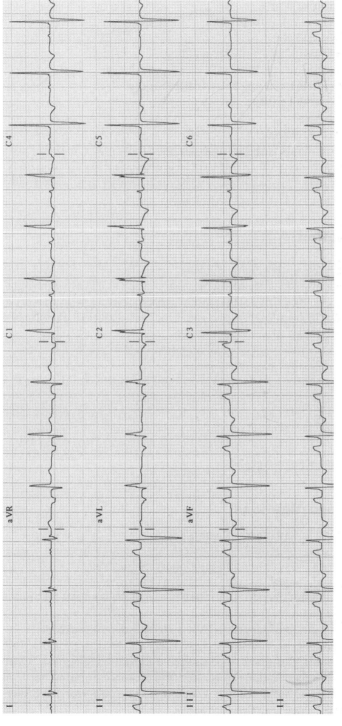

Fig. 20.2 12-lead resting electrocardiogram (EKG) from the same patient with Eisenmenger syndrome and a large VSD. Note extreme right axis deviation with right ventricular hypertrophy and first-degree heart block. T wave inversion across the left and precordial leads suggests possible ischemia.

- Sudden death (30%)
- Congestive heart failure (25%)
- Hemoptysis (15%)
- Other (30%) with a partial list including:
  - pregnancy;
  - perioperative following non-cardiac surgery;
  - infective endocarditis;
  - brain abscess;
  - non-cardiac causes.

While individuals with Eisenmenger syndrome may remain relatively stable for long periods of time, it is essential to appreciate that their hemodynamic state is very delicately balanced. This balance is easily upset, often with disastrous results.

Examination

- Central cyanosis with digital clubbing.
- Patients with a PDA may have normal-appearing nail beds on the right hand and cyanosis and clubbing of the nail beds of both feet and the left hand. (Venous blood shunts through the PDA and enters the aorta distal to the right subclavian artery.)
- Hypoxemia with resting oxygen saturation <90%.
- Lungs are usually clear.
- Elevated pulmonary artery pressures: right ventricle heave, palpable P_2, right-sided S_4, and occasionally a pulmonary ejection click.
- Murmurs likely to be heard include a high-pitched diastolic decrescendo murmur of pulmonic insufficiency and a holosystolic murmur of tricuspid regurgitation. Murmurs related to the defects connecting the systemic and pulmonary circulations are not usually heard.

Useful investigations

An evaluation to confirm the diagnosis shows:
- presence of a congenital heart defect large enough to cause a significant shunt between the systemic and pulmonary circulations;
- elevated pulmonary vascular resistance (>800 dyne-sec cm^{-5} or >10 units);
- reversal of or bidirectional shunting between the systemic and pulmonary circulations leading to hypoxemia;
- lack of significant reduction in PVR with oxygen or nitric oxide.

Transthoracic echo, transesophageal echo, CT, MRI, and cardiac catheterization are modalities that can be used to establish the diagnosis. Open lung biopsy is infrequently done to confirm the presence of pulmonary vascular occlusive disease, but if needed, it should only be performed at centers with ongoing experience with this technique.

It is important to be certain that the diagnosis of Eisenmenger syndrome is correct. One does not want to miss the opportunity to identify individuals who have reversibility of their pulmonary vascular disease that may enable a surgical repair of the defect. The case can be made that before attaching the diagnosis, a cardiac catheterization is performed to establish that the PVR is elevated and unresponsive to administration of oxygen or nitric oxide.

Catheter and surgical management

Once Eisenmenger physiology has developed, catheter or surgical interventions have a limited role in management. Surgery to repair the underlying congenital anomaly is not recommended, for two reasons: the risk of surgery is exceedingly high, and those that survive the surgery have increased mortality. Heart–lung transplantation is an option, but long waits (years) for eventual transplantation make the timing of this decision difficult. In some instances, lung transplantation with repair of the intracardiac defect may be an option. Lung transplantation has the advantage of better donor availability, a shorter waiting period, and avoidance of problems associated with heart transplantation (vasculopathy and rejection). The following may lead one to consider these options:
- progressive deterioration of functional class;
- recurrent syncope;
- refractory right heart failure;
- supraventricular tachyarrhythmias;
- worsening hypoxemia.

Complications

The chronic hypoxemia adversely affects multiple organs as follows.

- Cardiac:
  - progressive heart failure;
  - arrhythmias (atrial flutter/fibrillation);
  - angina;
  - syncope;
  - paradoxical emboli;
  - endocarditis;
  - progressive pulmonary artery enlargement.
- Hematopoietic:
  - erythrocytosis;
  - hyperviscosity syndrome;
  - iron deficiency;
  - neutropenia and thrombocytopenia;
  - bleeding disorder.
- Pulmonary:
  - hemoptysis;

  – intra-pulmonary bleeding;
  – pulmonary artery thrombosis.
- Central nervous system:
  – stroke/TIA;
  – brain abscess.
- Renal:
  – proteinuria and hematuria;
  – mildly elevated creatinine;
  – progressive renal failure.
- Metabolic:
  – hyperuricemia and gout;
  – hyperbilirubinemia and gallstones;
  – nephrolithiasis.

Expected abnormalities

A number of abnormal findings are expected in individuals with Eisenmenger syndrome and should not raise undue concern unless they represent a significant change from past values.

- Oxygen saturation at rest usually ranges in the lower to mid-80s. If checked shortly after exertion (even walking into the examination room), it will be lower (mid 70% range). The baseline value should be established after a few minutes of absolute rest.
- Hematocrit is usually high and may be as high as the 70s.
- Platelet count is low, usually 100–150,000 range, but values are often below 100,000.
- White blood cell count can be at the lower limits or normal or slightly reduced.
- INR and APTT are mildly prolonged.
- Uric acid and bilirubin are elevated.
- Proteinuria is present, usually less than 1 gram/24 hours. This is glomerular in origin and related to the hypoxemia. Mildly elevated serum creatinine and hematuria can also be found. These renal abnormalities usually do not warrant further evaluation, but it is important to avoid drugs or procedures that may further impair renal function.

Hypoxemia: while it seems obvious that inhaled oxygen would help, no studies show a mortality or morbidity benefit from chronic oxygen administration. Inhaled oxygen can be used if the patient feels a benefit exists (reduced dyspnea, reduced fatigue, improved sleep), however, the adverse effects of mucosal dryness leading to mucous bleeding and the cumbersome equipment cause most patients to chose not to chronically use oxygen.

Hyperviscosity syndrome: this syndrome entails a specific set of symptoms classified as mild, moderate or severe, and this includes headaches, altered mental status, visual disturbances, tinnitus, dizziness, paresthesias, myalgias and fatigue.

  The basis for this syndrome is increased viscosity of blood leading to decreased flow and oxygen delivery to tissues. Viscosity is affected by the concentration of red blood cells (RBCs) and their deformability. A high hematocrit alone may not cause these symptoms and may not require any intervention. Thus, an individual can be asymptomatic at a hematocrit >70%. If symptoms of hyperviscosity do occur at a hematocrit below 65%, blood viscosity is increased due to reduced RBC deformability rather than excessive erythrocytosis. The major etiology for reduced deformity is thought to be iron deficiency which causes RBCs to change from deformable biconcave disks to more rigid microspheres. Blood loss related to phlebotomy, hemoptysis, epistaxis and menses are common causes of iron deficiency.

The following are important considerations in individuals with symptoms suggestive of hyperviscosity syndrome.

• High hematocrit in the absence of symptoms does not require phlebotomy.

• Exclude dehydration as a cause if the hematocrit has increased.

• Exclude iron deficiency as a cause of symptoms. If present, treat with low-dose oral iron, monitoring hematocrit response.

• Phlebotomy may be appropriate if symptoms are severe and none of the above factors apply. The goal of phlebotomy is to treat the symptoms of the hyperviscosity syndrome and not to obtain a specific hematocrit. Prompt relief of symptoms after the phlebotomy confirms that hyperviscosity was the likely etiology. If the symptoms do not resolve promptly, consider other alternative causes and do not repeat the phlebotomy. In reality, phlebotomy is rarely needed. If needed, the protocol for phlebotomy is as follows.

– Withdraw 200–500 ml of blood over 30–45 minutes.

– Follow with equivalent volume replacement using isotonic saline.

– Monitor heart rate and blood pressure during and after phlebotomy, avoiding hypotension. Check orthostatic pressures before the individual is discharged.

– Prevent iron deficiency by giving oral iron if needed.

– The duration of beneficial effect is variable.

Bleeding: individuals are at risk of bleeding from the relatively benign easy bruising to life-threatening massive intra-pulmonary hemorrhage and hemoptysis. Mild increases in INR and aPTT are present due to decreased levels of factors V, VII, VIII and X, thrombocytopenia, platelet dysfunction and increased fibrinolytic activity. Most bleeding is, however, minor, involves the mucocutaneous tissues, and responds to conservative management. Antiplatelet agents (aspirin, non-steroidal agents) should be avoided. Significant bleeding can be treated with vitamin K, fresh frozen plasma, platelets or cryoprecipitate. A phlebotomy may improve platelet function, increase platelet count and improve various coagulation abnormalities, but the mechanism for this is unclear. A phlebotomy can be considered prior to elective surgery to decrease the risk of bleeding.

Hemoptysis: although most episodes are mild and self-limiting, hemoptysis may be a life-threatening event. Bleeding can occur from bronchial or pulmonary arteries, aorto-pulmonary collaterals, or infarcted or damaged lung tissue. Management includes:

• bed rest with low threshold for hospitalization;

- chest radiography and CT scan to determine extent of hemorrhage;
- monitoring of blood count and oxygen saturation;
- bronchoscopy not usually indicated;
- embolization of culprit vessels identified by pulmonary angiography.

Cerebrovascular and other embolic events: a paradox of the Eisenmenger syndrome is that both a bleeding and a thrombotic diathesis are present. Neurologic events do occur, but at a surprisingly low level. Mechanisms include hemorrhage, emboli and infection with formation of a cerebral abscess.

Risk factors for embolic events are:
- iron deficiency, the major risk factor for cerebrovascular events. Avoiding phlebotomies and correcting iron deficiency are two essential strategies to reduce the risk of emboli;
- atrial fibrillation;
- hypertension;
- venous disease of the legs with paradoxical embolus.

Initiation of anticoagulation therapy to prevent further embolic events in individuals with Eisenmenger syndrome is a difficult decision, since bleeding is a major problem. The indications should be strong. The risk–benefit ratio of aspirin or warfarin needs to be considered in each patient. See Chapter 5 for further discussion of this complex issue.

Hyperuricemia and gout: in the adult patient with cyanosis, hyperuricemia is due to increased absorption of uric acid rather than increased production. Uric acid nephrolithiasis can occur.
- Asymptomatic hyperuricemia does not need treatment.
- Symptomatic hyperuricemia (gout) can be treated with:
  - colchicine, steroids, or both for the acute episode;
  - probenecid, sulfinpyrazone and allopurinol, all of which lower uric acid levels and may be used for prevention of recurrences;
  - salsalate (a nonacetylated anti-inflammatory analog of aspirin, with no effect on platelets) for pain. Try to avoid aspirin and other nonsteroidal anti-inflammatory drugs.

Arthralgias: arthralgias can also be caused by hypertrophic osteoarthropathy. This is due to local cell proliferation and new osseous formation with periostitis. Megakaryocytes released from the bone marrow bypass the lungs due to the right-to-left shunt and lodge in the capillaries of the bones. They induce the release of platelet-derived growth factor that promotes the new bone growth. Arthralgias of the knees and ankles are commonly noted. This is treated symptomatically with salsalate.

Pulmonary hypertension: pulmonary vasodilator agents such as prostacyclin analogs, endothelin antagonists and phosphodiesterase inhibitors have been found to reduce pulmonary vascular resistance and improve functional capacity in idiopathic (primary) and secondary pulmonary hypertension. Although the long-term prognosis for individuals with Eisenmenger syndrome is better than for those with idiopathic pulmonary hypertension, the histopathologic appearance of the pulmonary vasculature is similar in the two groups. This has led to the cautious use of these pulmonary vasodilator agents in the Eisenmenger syndrome patient. Since placebo-controlled trials are not available, the eventual role of these agents in treating individuals with an unrestricted defect and the potential for right-to-left shunting has not been established. However, the possibility of improving morbidity and mortality in the Eisenmenger patient with these medications is exciting. Limited data cite some individuals so responsive to these agents that surgical correction of the defect was possible. Alternatively, in patients with progressive heart failure, these agents have been used as part of a bridge to transplantation. Chapter 22 provides further information about treatment of pulmonary hypertension.

Late outcomes

A large variation in life expectancy exists for individuals with Eisenmenger syndrome. Reports that include pediatric patients found an average age at death in the 25–35 years range. Alternatively, mean survival in an adult population is in the 50–55 years range. Variables that are associated with increased mortality are:
- younger age at presentation;
- supraventricular arrhythmias;
- poor functional class;
- right ventricular hypertrophy on EKG or echo.

Required follow-up

These are some of the most complicated patients to manage and should be followed every 6–12 months by a cardiologist experienced in this unique pathophysiology. Almost any perturbation has the potential to upset the delicate hemodynamic balance, with a potentially disastrous outcome. Routine follow-up includes:

- clinical evaluation, including arterial saturation by transcutaneous oximetry;
- checking for hyperviscosity syndrome;
- checking hematocrit and iron status;
- checking for bleeding problems, especially excessive or prolonged menses;
- changes in functional capacity;
- occurrence of arrhythmias;
- reminding patient to avoid dehydration and extremes of exertion;
- reminding patient to avoid smoking;
- reminding patient to avoid pregnancy and discussion of birth control issues;
- reminding patient about endocarditis prophylaxis;
- reminding patient to consult physician regarding any new medications prescribed or procedures recommended;

• yearly laboratory work (FBC, ferritin, clotting parameters, multichem panel), chest radiography and EKG (Fig. 20.1). Echocardiographic studies are needed less frequently in stable individuals.

Endocarditis prophylaxis
Endocarditis prophylaxis at a high-risk level is recommended.

Exercise
While comfortable at rest, exercise capacity is markedly reduced in cyanotic individuals. Obvious problems include:
• increased right-to-left shunting, causing worsening hypoxemia;
• constrained blood flow through the lungs, so oxygen delivery does not increase;
• further decrease in venous blood saturation as peripheral oxygen extraction increases. This further reduces oxygen saturation;
• development of respiratory acidosis as shunting increases, since CO_2 is not removed from the shunted blood;
• increase in ventilation above that expected for any given level of oxygen consumption, leading to the sensation of dyspnea.

Individuals can usually perform most activities of daily living, but easily become tired. In addition, they are encouraged to perform light exertion as tolerated, avoiding extremes of exertion. Exertion that causes profound dyspnea, light-headedness or syncope should be avoided.

Residing at or traveling to high altitude (>5000 feet or 1500 m above sea level) will worsen hypoxemia and further limit exercise capacity. In contrast, commercial airline travel is usually safe (see Travel section in Chapter 6). Inflight oxygen is not usually required, but can be made available during a flight by advance arrangement with the airline if an individual requires it.

Pregnancy and contraception
Women with Eisenmenger syndrome should avoid pregnancy. If one presents pregnant, early termination is recommended; it is less risky than continuation of the pregnancy. The reason for these strong statements is that pregnancy causes significant maternal and fetal morbidity and mortality in women with cyanosis and pulmonary vascular disease. Maternal mortality is 30–45%, with death occurring during delivery or within several weeks postpartum. Deaths are commonly due to:
• thromboembolism (44%);
• hypovolemia (25%);
• pre-eclampsia (18%);
• worsening heart failure;
• progressive hypoxemia.

The fetus also fares poorly. Risks include:
• spontaneous abortion and stillbirth (20–40%);
• premature delivery (50%);

- intrauterine growth retardation (30%).

If the woman desires to continue a pregnancy despite being informed of the extreme risks, close observation by an experienced group of obstetricians, anesthesiologists and cardiologists familiar with Eisenmenger syndrome is recommended. A vaginal delivery with adequate pain control and a shortened second stage of labor are recommended. This approach may be less risky than a cesarean delivery. The latter may be considered for obstetric indications. Some advocate hospitalization at 25–30 weeks with close monitoring until delivery occurs spontaneously or is electively induced. Since death frequently occurs postpartum, continued observation in the hospital for 1–3 weeks has been advocated (see Chapter 3).

Another area of uncertainty is whether anticoagulation during pregnancy decreases the risk of death from thromboembolism. Some advocate routine use of subcutaneous heparin starting at 20 weeks with an aPTT 6 hours after injection of >2 times control. The heparin is discontinued several hours prior to delivery. Some recommend continuing full anticoagulation with warfarin for 1–2 months postpartum. Unfortunately, no data are available to support or refute these approaches.

Prevention of pregnancy should be addressed in women of childbearing age.
- Sterilization is the surest way to prevent a pregnancy. This can be done by laparoscopic techniques with a small risk, or by the newer technique of transvaginal tubal obstruction with even lower risk.
- Oral contraceptives carry risks of thromboembolism and worsening heart failure due to fluid retention. While these risks are important to consider, they are much less than that of a pregnancy.
- Barrier methods (condoms, diaphragms) are less desirable due to a high failure rate (see Chapter 3).

Non-cardiac surgery in Eisenmenger patients is a significant issue as it carries a high morbidity and mortality risk (up to 19%). Surgery should be avoided when possible, but is commonly needed for acute cholecystitis (due to bilirubin stone formation from the hyperbilirubinemia). Necessary operations should be done in a center familiar with the high risks of performing surgery on these patients.

Perioperative morbidity and mortality

The mortality and morbidity are related to:
- sudden fall in SVR leading to worsening hypoxemia due to progressive right-to-left shunting;
- hypovolemia and dehydration which are poorly tolerated and worsen right-to-left shunting;
- excessive bleeding;
- perioperative arrhythmias;
- thrombophlebitis/deep vein thrombosis/paradoxical emboli.

Techniques of risk reduction

- Surgery should be done at a center experienced in congenital heart disease.
- An experienced cardiac anesthesiologist should be present.
- Avoid prolonged fasting without fluid replacement prior to surgery.
- Air filter for all intravenous lines.
- A central pulmonary artery catheter is not indicated, but a good peripheral or central IV is helpful.
- Meticulous attention to bleeding and blood loss.
- Postoperative monitoring in an intensive care unit setting.
- Systemic arterial hypotension should be treated quickly and aggressively with intravenous fluids, blood transfusion, or an alpha adrenergic agent.
- Early ambulation to reduce the risk of emboli from deep vein thrombosis.

Key clinical points

- Survival of patients with Eisenmenger syndrome into adulthood is common.
- Their medical issues are complex and are best taken care of by cardiologists who understand their physiology and the medical issues involved.
- These individuals are in a delicate balance that can be easily upset leading to disastrous results. Important risks to be aware of are:
  - pregnancy (contraindicated);
  - non-cardiac surgery (morbidity and mortality risk);
  - dehydration;
  - bleeding or hemorrhage, especially intrapulmonary;
  - antiplatelet drugs that increase the risk of bleeding;
  - drugs that reduce systemic vascular resistance (increase shunting);
  - anemia and iron deficiency;
  - air emboli from intravenous lines;
  - cardiac catheterization;
  - pulmonary infections.
- The role of vasodilator agents to reduce pulmonary vascular resistance in the Eisenmenger patients is evolving. Although not yet adequately studied, it has the potential to significantly improve their overall morbidity and mortality and improve functional class.

Further reading

Amish N & Warnes CA (1996) Cebrovascular events in adult patients with cyanotic congenital heart disease. *Journal of the American College of Cardiology*, **28**, 768–772.

Ammash NM, Connolly HM, Abel M & Warnes CA. Noncardiac surgery in Eisenmenger syndrome. *Journal of the American College of Cardiology*, **33**, 222–227.

Cantor WJ, Harrison DA, Moussadji JS, *et al.* (1999) Determinants of survival and length of survival in adults with Eisenmenger syndrome. *American Journal of Cardiology*, **84**, 677–681.

Daliento L, Somerville J, Presbitero P, *et al.* (1998) Eisenmenger syndrome. Factors relating to deterioration and death. *European Heart Journal*, **19**, 1845–1855.

Eisenmenger V (1897) Die angeborenen Defekte der Kammerscheidewand des Herzen. (Congenital defects of the ventricular septum). *Zeitschrift fur Klinische Medizin*, **32** (Suppl), 1–28.

Niwa K, Perloff JK, Kaplan S, Child JS & Miner PD (1999) Eisenmenger syndrome in adults: Ventricular septal defect, truncus arteriosus, univentricular heart. *Journal of the American College of Cardiology*, **34**, 223–232.

Perloff JK, Marelli AJ & Miner PD (1993) Risk of stroke in adults with cyanotic congenital heart disease. *Circulation*, **98**, 1954–1959.

Vongpatanasin W, Brickner E, Hillis D & Lange RA (1998) The Eisenmenger syndrome in adults. *Annals of Internal Medicine*, **128**, 745–755.

Wood P (1958) The Eisenmenger syndrome or pulmonary hypertension with reversed central shunt. *British Medical Journal*, **2**, 701–709 and 755–762.

CHAPTER 21

Other Lesions

Common arterial trunk

Definition and natural history

Common arterial trunk, also known as truncus arteriosus, is an uncommon lesion consisted of a single great artery (arterial trunk) coming off the ventricular mass. There is always a large ventricular septal defect (VSD). The pulmonary arteries in turn come off the ascending aorta, either through a common stem or independently (Fig. 21.1a). There is no direct communication, therefore, between the pulmonary trunk and the right ventricle. The truncal valve is often dysplastic with three or more leaflets and may be regurgitant and/or stenotic from birth. The degree of valval deformity is one of the key determinants of outcome.

Therapy is surgical, involving VSD closure and conduit anastomosis between the right ventricle and the pulmonary arteries (which themselves may need unifocalization procedures). If not operated during the first year of life,

(a) Common arterial trunk   (b) Aortopulmonary window

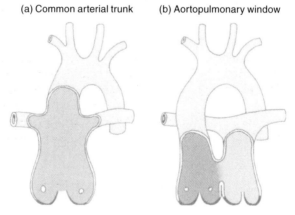

Fig. 21.1 (a) Common arterial trunk. Note the single exit from the heart via the common arterial valve and trunk, giving rise to the right and left pulmonary arteries (from the ascending aorta). Alternatively, the pulmonary arteries may arise from a common stem from the ascending aorta before dividing to right and left, or occasionally one of them may arise from the underside of the aorta. The truncal valve may have more than three leaflets, is often dysplastic, causing stenosis and or regurgitation and is a major determinant of long-term outcome. (b) Aortopulmonary window. Note the two exits from the heart with a normal aortic and pulmonary valve and a large nonrestrictive communication between the two arterial trunks (window) at relatively close proximity to the semilunar valves. Patients require early repair to avoid irreversible pulmonary vascular disease.

most patients will develop irreversible pulmonary vascular disease and would be deemed inoperable thereafter.

Approximately one-third of patients with common arterial trunk have Di-George syndrome. This needs to be addressed with the patient and the family as it has important genetic implications. Most cases of DiGeorge syndrome are sporadic, but the risk of recurrence is 50% and these patients are also at risk of early psychiatric disease.

Older patients are likely to require further surgery to replace the right ventricular to pulmonary artery conduit.

Late complications

- Right ventricular to pulmonary artery conduit stenosis or regurgitation.
- Branch pulmonary artery stenoses.
- Residual VSD.
- Truncal valve regurgitation or stenosis, or prosthetic valve dysfunction when the truncal valve has been replaced.
- Myocardial ischemia due to coronary artery anomalies.
- Progressive aortic root dilatation which may lead to neo-aortic valve incompetence.
- Ventricular dysfunction which may result from multiple surgical interventions, conduit dysfunction and/or myocardial ischemia.
- Progressive pulmonary vascular disease.
- Arrhythmias and sudden cardiac death.

Pregnancy

Successful pregnancy and delivery are possible in patients with repaired common arterial trunk. Given the high incidence of chromosome 22q11 deletion (DiGeorge syndrome), chromosomal analysis using the FISH test (fluorescent in situ hybridization) should be offered to all women with the condition who are contemplating pregnancy. All patients should have pre-pregnancy counseling and careful follow-up during pregnancy by a specialist cardiologist.

Endocarditis

All patients should practice endocarditis prophylaxis for life.

Exercise

Advice regarding the intensity of exercise will depend on the outcome of repair, the severity of residual lesions (conduit stenosis, truncal valve function, etc.), the state of ventricular function and the presence or not of pulmonary hypertension.

Aortopulmonary window

Definition and natural history

Aortopulmonary (AP) window is a rare lesion that can mimic patent arterial duct (Fig. 21.1b). It is a direct communication between ascending aorta and pulmonary artery resulting from an incomplete division of the embryonic common arterial trunk. Usually, the defect is large and, therefore, the likelihood of pulmonary hypertension being established in the adult patient is high, unless closure took place early in childhood. About 10% of AP windows are relatively small and, therefore, not susceptible to developing early pulmonary hypertension. Aortopulmonary windows are commonly associated with other cardiac lesions such as VSD, tetralogy of Fallot, subaortic stenosis, atrial septal defect or patent ductus arteriosus and, therefore, can be easily overlooked.

Patients with an AP window present either with congestive heart failure early in the course of the disease or, if pulmonary hypertension has developed, with cyanosis. Occasionally, when the AP window is relatively small, they can present with a continuous murmur and signs of left heart dilatation due to volume overload. Unless irreversible pulmonary vascular disease has developed, patients should undergo timely surgical repair. Catheter device closure has also been reported.

Observational points

- Confirm the absence of residual AP communication.
- Assess associated lesions, if present.
- Assess left ventricular size and function.
- Exclude pulmonary hypertension.
- Exclude important supravalvar pulmonary stenosis, when a 'tunnel type' of surgical repair has been performed.

Pregnancy, endocarditis and exercise

The same principles as for common arterial trunk apply. However, the risk of DiGeorge syndrome and therefore of recurrence of heart disease is lower. Pregnancy and exercise are largely determined by the degree of pulmonary hypertension, if present. Most patients warrant lifelong endocarditis prophylaxis, because of the very common associated lesions.

Sinus of Valsalva aneurysms

Definition and natural history

Sinus of Valsalva aneurysm is defined as dilatation or enlargement of one of the aortic sinuses between the aortic valve annulus and the sinotubular junction (Fig. 21.2). The morphology of sinus of Valsalva aneurysms can vary from a small isolated enlargement of the aortic sinus (usually the right sinus) to an extended finger-like projection from the body or apex of the sinus. This tubular protrusion may extend into the adjacent structures, causing a variety of clinical sequelae. The right coronary sinus is the commonest site for aneursym formation (65–85%). VSDs are a very common association.

The diagnosis is made echocardiographically.

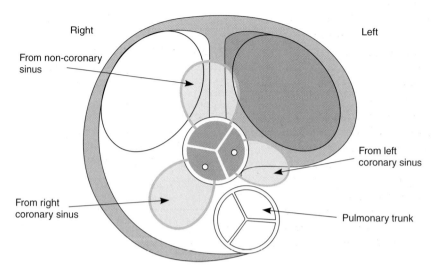

Fig. 21.2 Aneurysms of the sinus of Valsalva. Various origins and positions of aneurysms of Valsalva (when heart base is seen from above).

Ruptured sinus of Valsalva aneurysms may occasionally present dramatically with sudden hemodynamic collapse, or chronically, depending on the size and site of the rupture.

The most common 'receiving' chamber:
• right ventricle (90%);
• right atrium (10%);
• left atrium (2–3%).
  Free perforation into the pericardium is almost invariably associated with fatal cardiac tamponade, but is rare.

Cardiac arrest and sudden cardiac death can occur if the rupture causes acute disruption of a coronary ostium. Rupture with acute aortic cusp distortion results in aortic valvular insufficiency and myocardial still phenomenon. Chest pain, cough and breathlessness are often the first features combined with the onset of a loud continuous 'to-and-fro' murmur due to the fistula. Ruptured sinus of Valsalva aneurysms should be surgically repaired without delay.

Pregnancy, endocarditis and exercise
As in patients with Marfan syndrome, those with known unruptured sinus of Valsalva aneurysms should be cautioned before embarking on pregnancy. Indeed, pregnancy may be the decisive factor for expediting surgical repair. Exercise should be determined by the hemodynamic status of the patient, although extreme isometric exercise should be discouraged. All patients warrant lifelong endocarditis prophylaxis.

Late complications of sinus of Valsalva aneurysms

Unruptured	Ruptured
Compressive • Right ventricular outflow tract (RVOT) obstruction • Obstruction of coronary ostium: ischemia, arrhythmia • Left ventricular outflow obstruction (rare) • Arrhythmia: RVOT ventricular tachycardia • Atrioventricular block *Embolic* • Peripheral embolism • TIA *Infective endocarditis*	• Cardiac tamponade • Left-to-right shunt • Acute heart failure • Acute valvular regurgitation (aortic; tricuspid) • Acute disruption of coronary artery • Septal 'mass' • Arrhythmia • Infective endocarditis

With permission from Swan L (2003) Chapter on Sinus of Valsalva Aneurysms. In: *Diagnosis and Management of Adult Congenital Heart Disease* (eds Gatzoulis, Webb and Daubeney), pp. 239–243; Elsevier, Philadelphia, PA.

Cor triatriatum

Cor triatriatum is a rare congenital cardiac anomaly in which the common pulmonary venous chamber is separated from the true left atrium by a fibro-muscular septum (Fig. 21.3). Approximately 70–80% of cases of cor triatriatum are associated with other cardiac defects, secundum atrial septal defect being the most common.

The age at presentation and clinical symptoms relate directly to the degree of pulmonary venous obstruction. Patients with a very restrictive membrane in general present early with symptoms of pulmonary hypertension. A second group of patients present in adulthood with atrial fibrillation and/or throm-boembolic events such as TIA or stroke. These patients have a dilated proximal

Normal Cor triatriatum

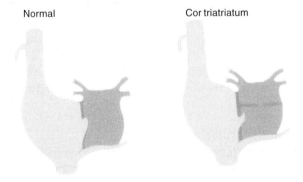

Fig. 21.3 Cor triatriatum. This is seen as a membrane dividing the left atrium into the proximal (pulmonary venous) and distal chamber in the right panel, compared to the normal heart (left panel). Note the commonly coexisting atrial septal defect, opening in this case into the distal left atrial chamber.

left atrial compartment with dilated pulmonary veins, both of which represent the source of atrial fibrillation and clot formation. Finally, there is a third group of patients with no or minimal obstruction of flow at the level of the cor triatriatum, the diagnosis being a coincidental echocardiographic finding. With the exception of the latter group, patients should undergo elective surgical excision of the membrane and repair of associated defects, anticipating a good outcome.

Dilatation of the membrane, either intraoperatively or with percutaneous balloon catheterization, has been reported but is unlikely to result in permanent relief of symptoms.

Pregnancy, endocarditis and exercise

Following successful repair of cor triatriatum and, provided that there is no residual pulmonary hypertension, there should be no contraindications to pregnancy (which in turn should carry a very low risk). For postoperative patients, normal physical activities should be encouraged, and unless there are residual hemodynamic lesions there is no need for endocarditis prophylaxis.

Atrial isomerism (heterotaxia)

Right and left isomerism means equal parts and refers to duplication or predominance of thoracic and abdominal organs exhibiting rightness or leftness, respectively. Isomerism is thus applicable to atria, bronchi, lungs, spleen, etc. (Fig. 21.4).

Left atrial isomerism (also called polysplenia) is associated with multiple spleens. Right atrial isomerism (asplenia syndrome) is associated with small or poorly functional spleen(s), the latter being a left-sided organ. Patients with left or right atrial isomerism, apart from the presence of two morphologically left or right atria, almost universally have additional intracardiac defects.

Complex cardiac anatomy with 'single ventricle physiology' is particularly common in patients with right atrial isomerism. For these patients the Fontan route is the main surgical option available.

Conduction abnormalities are also common in atrial isomerism and contribute to morbidity and mortality. There are other important non-cardiac manifestations affecting outcomes in these patients that general physicians should be aware of so that appropriate measures can be taken. A typical example is functional asplenia in patients with right atrial isomerism, predisposing them to pneumococcal infections. Such patients would benefit from chronic oral penicillin therapy and periodic immunization.

In general, all patients with isomerism should be managed in tertiary adult congenital heart disease centers.

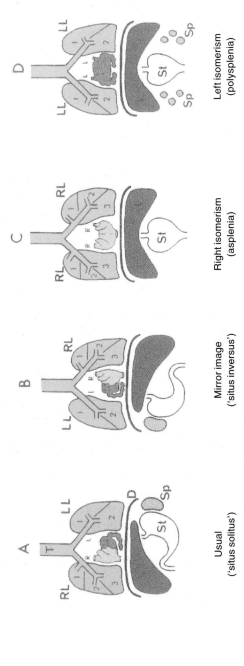

Fig. 21.4 Right and left atrial isomerism (asplenia and polysplenia syndromes, respectively). Atrial, bronchial and abdominal arrangements. Usual or situs solitus (left panel, A), mirror image or situs inversus (left middle panel, B), right atrial isomerism or asplenia syndrome (right middle panel, C) and left atrial isomerism or polysplenia syndrome (right panel, D). R, morphological right atrium; L, morphological left atrium; T, trachea; RL, right lung; LL, left lung; St, stomach; L, liver; Sp, spleen.

Right atrial isomerism	Left atrial isomerism
Common cardiac lesions	*Common cardiac lesions*
Total anomalous pulmonary veins	Interrupted inferior vena cava (with azygous
Atrioventricular (AV) septal defect	continuation)
Transposition of great arteries or double outlet	Partial anomalous pulmonary veins
right ventricle	Atrial and/or ventricular septal defect
Pulmonary stenosis or atresia	Double outlet right ventricle
Airway morphology	*Airway morphology*
Bilateral trilobar lungs	Bilateral bilobar lungs
Short main bronchi	Long main bronchi
Other	*Other*
Functional asplenia with immunodeficiency	Polysplenia
Malrotation of bowel	Malrotation of bowel
Howell-Jolly bodies in blood film	Biliary atresia
Dual sinus or AV node	Absent sinus node (with ectopic atrial node or
	wandering pacemaker) and/or complete heart
	block

Further reading

Anderson RH, Devine W & Uemura H (1995) Diagnosis of heterotaxy syndrome. *Circulation*, **91**, 906–908.

Bertolini A, Dalmonte P, Bava GL, Moretti R, Cervo G & Marasini M (1994) Aortopulmonary septal defects. A review of the literature and report of ten cases. *Journal of Cardiovascular Surgery*, **35**(3), 207–213.

Gilljam T, McCrindle BW, Smallhorn JF, Williams WG & Freedom RM (2000) Outcomes of left atrial isomerism over a 28-year period at a single institution. *Journal of the American College of Cardiology*, **36**, 908–916.

Hashmi A, Abu-Sulaiman R, McCrindle BW, Smallhorn JF, Williams WG & Freedom RM (1998) Management and outcome of right atrial isomerism: a 26 year experience. *Journal of the American College of Cardiology*, **31**, 1120–1126.

Kirklin JW & Barrett-Boyes BG (1993) Truncus arteriosus. In: *Cardiac Surgery*, 2nd edn, p. 1140. Churchill Livingstone.

Marcelletti C, McGoon DC & Mair DD (1976) The natural history of truncus arteriosus. *Circulation*, **54**, 108.

Takach TJ, Reul GJ, Duncan JM, *et al.* (1999) Sinus of Valsalva aneurysm or fistula: management and outcome. *Annals of Thoracic Surgery*, **68**, 1573–1577.

Tulloh RM & Rigby ML (1997) Transcatheter umbrella closure of aorto-pulmonary window. *Heart*, **77**, 479–480.

Van Son JA, Danielson GK, Schaff HV, *et al.* (1993) Cor triatriatum: diagnosis, operative approach, and late results. *Mayo Clinic Proceedings*, **68**, 854–859.

Williams JM, De Leeuw M, Black MD, Freedom RF, Williams WG & McCrindle BW (1999) Factors associated with outcomes of persistent truncus arteriosus. *Journal of the American College of Cardiology*, **34**, 545–553.

CHAPTER 22

Pulmonary Hypertension

Pulmonary hypertension is defined as any elevation of mean pulmonary artery pressure greater than 25 mmHg at rest or 30 mmHg with exercise. This is due to either an increase in flow through the pulmonary vascular bed, as typically in congenital heart disease, or to a reduction in caliber of pulmonary arterioles secondary to a number of different mechanisms.

Causes of pulmonary hypertension

Pulmonary arterial hypertension
• Primary pulmonary hypertension (or so-called idiopathic, no specific cause found)
• Collagen vascular disease
• Congenital heart defects (includes Eisenmenger physiology)
• Portal hypertension
• HIV infection
• Drugs/toxins
• Appetite suppressants

Pulmonary venous hypertension
• Left-sided valvular heart disease
• Hypertrophic, restrictive and or dilated cardiomyopathy
• Left atrial myxoma
• Extrinsic compression of central pulmonary veins
• Pulmonary veno-occlusive disease

Pulmonary hypertension associated with respiratory disorders
• Chronic obstructive pulmonary disease
• Interstitial lung disease
• Sleep apnea
• Alveolar hypoventilation disorders
• Chronic exposure to high altitude
• Neonatal lung disease

Pulmonary hypertension due to chronic thrombotic and/or embolic disease
• Thromboembolic obstruction of proximal pulmonary arteries
• Obstruction of distal pulmonary arteries due to:

- pulmonary embolism (thrombus, tumor, parasites, foreign material);
- in situ thrombosis;
- sickle cell disease.

Pulmonary hypertension due to disorders directly affecting the pulmonary vasculature

- Inflammatory due to:
  - schistosomiasis;
  - sarcoidosis;
  - pulmonary capillary hemangiomatosis.

A number of triggering factors (Fig. 22.1) are thought to be responsible, and in many cases there seems to be a genetic predisposition to developing pulmonary hypertension.

Ultimately, chronic pulmonary hypertension (PHT) is associated with intimal thickening of pulmonary arterioles and medial hypertrophy in larger

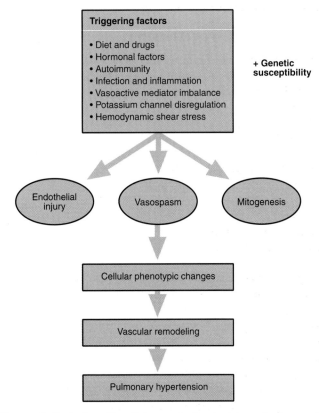

Fig. 22.1 Diagramatic illustration of the etiology and pathophysiology of pulmonary hypertension. With permission from Mikhail GW & Yacoub MH (2003) in Gatzoulis, Webb and Daubeney (eds), *Diagnosis and Management of Adult Congenital Heart Disease*, Elsevier, Philadephia, PA.

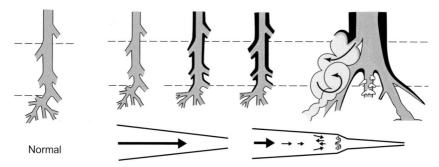

Normal

Fig. 22.2 Evolution of pulmonary vascular disease in the young, showing the early reduction in number of arteries, the increase in muscularity, and development of intimal proliferation. Blood flow patterns change from laminar to turbulent with disease progression. With permission from Haworth SG (2002) *Heart*, **88**, 658–664.

arteries (Fig. 22.2). Vessels may be totally occluded by the endothelial proliferation and/or secondary intravascular thrombosis.

Primary pulmonary hypertension

This is a rare disease with an annual incidence of approximately 1 per 200,000–1,000,000 population. It is more common in young women. Endothelial dysfunction has been identified in primary pulmonary hypertension (PPH), either as a cause or effect. Lung biopsies have shown reduced expression of nitric oxide synthase, reduced levels of PGI_2 and increased endothelin-1, all contributing to hypertrophy and thrombus formation in the pulmonary microvasculature. Larger central vessels may also contain larger thrombus.

Clinical factors implicated include:

* chronic small pulmonary emboli;
* collagen vascular disease (association with Raynaud's phenomenon);
* scleroderma.

Symptoms and clinical signs

The onset of symptoms in PPH is usually subtle, with several years elapsing before the diagnosis is made. Common symptoms are as follows.

* *Exertional dyspnea*: patients with pulmonary hypertension tend to hyperventilate to compensate for arterial hypoxemia, which is a result of ventilation perfusion mismatch in the lung and a reduced cardiac output.
* *Syncope* is common (often exertional): pulmonary hypertensive patients have a reduced cardiac output and compromised left ventricular function. Hence, even a benign tachycardia can lead to systemic hypotension and hemodynamic syncope.
* *Angina*: patients have right ventricular ischemia.
* *Sudden cardiac death*: presumably arrhythmic. Rupture of central pulmonary arteries has also been reported.

The *physical signs* in patients with pulmonary hypertension are usually advanced at the time of presentation. They include:

- central cyanosis;
- prominent 'a' wave in JVP;
- right ventricular (RV) heave;
- palpable pulmonary artery pulsation;
- loud pulmonary component to the second heart sound (often palpable);
- third and fourth heart sound at late stages;
- diastolic murmur of pulmonary regurgitation (Graham Steell)/pansystolic murmur of tricuspid regurgitation;
- pulsatile hepatomegaly, ascites and peripheral pitting edema (late stage).

Useful investigations

Patients with a suspected diagnosis of PPH should be referred without delay to a specialized center, where the diagnosis can be confirmed and therapy initiated early when it is most likely to be of benefit. Appropriate screening for patients with suspected pulmonary hypertension is, therefore, imperative for early diagnosis and treatment.

- **EKG**: severe RV strain (T wave inversion in V1–V3), right axis deviation and incomplete or complete RBBB. Right ventricular hypertrophy. Usually in sinus rhythm with evidence of right atrial overload. PR interval often prolonged (reflecting right atrial enlargement).
- **Chest radiography** (Fig. 22.3): normal heart size (early stage) with dilated main and central pulmonary arteries, but pruned peripheral arteries. Lung peripheries look dark and oligemic.

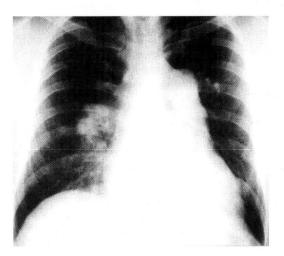

Fig. 22.3 Chest radiograph from a patient with primary pulmonary arterial hypertension. Note moderate to severe cardiomegaly and marked dilatation of central pulmonary arteries. The former suggests cardiac decompensation. Peripheral pulmonary artery 'prooning' is present, in contrast to radiographic appearance of patient with Eisenmenger physiology (Fig. 20.1a).

• **Echocardiography**: confirms PHT and RV hypertrophy. Pulmonary and tricuspid regurgitation are commonly present. Assess RV pressure from TR Doppler pressure gradients. Exclude occult left heart problems as a possible cause of PHT such as mitral or aortic valve disease, atrial myxoma, cor triatriatum, etc.

• **Cardiac catheterization**: remains the gold standard for establishing the diagnosis of primary PHT. Pulmonary hypertension is defined as an increase in mean pulmonary artery pressure >25 mmHg at rest or >30 mmHg during exercise. At cardiac catheterization, hemodynamic measurements of right heart pressures, cardiac output and mixed venous saturations and pulmonary vascular resistance (see Appendix for formula for shunt and pulmonary vascular resistance calculations) are carried out, as well as testing of acute vasodilator response (reversibility). Cardiac catheterization carries a low but definite risk.

• **Six-minute walk test**: useful for assessing the severity of symptoms in patients with pulmonary hypertension and monitoring individual patients and their response to therapy.

Management

Primary pulmonary hypertension remains a relentlessly progressive and fatal disease, with a mean survival from diagnosis of 2 to 3 years. However, new therapeutic modalities and a quest for establishing an early diagnosis are expected to convey a better outcome for many patients with this condition.

The main therapies are listed below.

• *Anticoagulation*: routine. Shown to improve survival.

• *Calcium antagonists*: high doses of long-acting drugs are needed, but only about 20% of patients will respond with a fall in pulmonary vascular resistance. A gradual increase in dose is advisable unless monitored with a Swan–Ganz catheter in situ. Typical doses needed: nifedipine 180–240 mg daily or diltiazem 720 mg daily. Systemic hypotension may be problematic. Responders have improved prognosis.

• *Domiciliary oxygen* may help patients who can still be managed at home.

• *Intravenous prostacyclin (epoprostenol)*: infusion via central lines. Shown to improve symptoms, hemodynamics and survival. Generally reserved for more severe or deteriorating cases when it may be used as a bridge to transplantation. Infusion dosing is performed with right heart catheterization. Start at 2 ng/kg/min, increasing by 2 ng/kg/min every 15 min. Increments are stopped when arterial pressure falls by 40%, or heart rate increases by 40%, or patient develops intolerant symptoms (nausea, vomiting, headache, etc.).

• *Subcutaneous prostacyclin*: heat-stable form of prostacyclin (Treprostinil) improves exercise capacity and pulmonary hemodynamics. There are problems, however, with injection site pain, which may limit its use.

• *Beraprost* is an oral prostacyclin analog which has been shown to have a vasodilator and antiplatelet activity similar to that of prostacyclin and is effective by oral administration.

• *Inhaled nitric oxide*: a selective pulmonary vasodilator, frequently used in the hospital setting for the acute reduction of pulmonary artery pressure in patients

with PPH. It may be of use for pregnant women with pulmonary arterial hypertension.
- *Bosentan*: an oral dual endothelin receptor antagonist, shown to be of benefit in pulmonary hypertension. Recent trials have shown improvement in pulmonary hemodynamics, exercise capacity and functional class. Bosentan is easy to administer and has an acceptable safety profile.
- *Sildenafil*: an inhibitor of cGMP-specific phosphodiesterase type 5, decreases the degradation of cyclic guanosine monophosphate (cGMP). Results in local release of nitric oxide and vasodilation.
- *Surgical treatment*
  - *Atrial septostomy:* shown to be of benefit in patients with recurrent syncope. By creating a right-to-left shunt at the atrial level, it is possible to decompress the right ventricle and improve left ventricular filling, thus maintaining cardiac output. However, there is a risk of severe oxygen desaturation and the procedure itself carries a significant risk.
  - *Thromboendartercetomy*: surgical removal of the organized thrombotic material for patients with chronic thromboembolic pulmonary hypertension, who have otherwise a poor prognosis. Operative mortality is usually less than 10% in big centers with good long-term results and a fall in pulmonary vascular resistance and improvement in right ventricular function.
  - *Heart and lung transplantation*: reserved for patients with progressive clinical deterioration despite medical therapy. With the continuing improvement in surgical techniques and rapid advances in immunosuppressive therapy, one-year survival for this challenging group of patients has reached 65–70%. Obliterative bronchiolitis, however, remains a major longer-term complication.

Further reading

Abenhaim L, Moride Y, Brenot F, *et al.* (1996) Appetite-suppressant drugs and the risk of primary pulmonary hypertension. International Primary Pulmonary Hypertension Study Group. *New England Journal of Medicine*, **335**(9), 609–616.

Barst RJ, Rubin LJ, Long WA, *et al.* (1996) A comparison of continuous intravenous epoprostenol (prostacyclin) with conventional therapy for primary pulmonary hypertension. The Primary Pulmonary Hypertension Study Group. *New England Journal of Medicine*, **334**(5), 296–302.

Channick RN, Simonneau G, Sitbon O, *et al.* (2001) Effects of the dual endothelin-receptor antagonist bosentan in patients with pulmonary hypertension: a randomised placebo-controlled study. *Lancet*, **358**, 1119–1123.

Gibbs JSR (2001) Recommendations on the management of pulmonary hypertension in clinical practice. *Heart*, **86** (Suppl) i11–i13.

McLaughlin VA, Genthner DE, Panella MM & Rich S (1998) Reduction in pulmonary vascular resistance with long-term epoprostenol (prostacyclin) therapy in primary pulmonary hypertension. *New England Journal of Medicine*, **338**, 273–277.

Mikhail G, Gibbs JSR, Richardson M, *et al.* (1997) An evaluation of nebulized prostacyclin in primary and secondary pulmonary hypertension. *European Heart Journal*, **18**, 1499–504.

Nagaya N, Uematsu M, Okano Y, *et al.* (1999) Effect of orally active prostacyclin analogue on survival of outpatients with primary pulmonary hypertension. *Journal of the American College of Cardiology*, **34**, 1188–1192.

Prasad S, Wilkinson J & Gatzoulis MA (2000) Sildenafil in primary pulmonary hypertension. *New England Journal of Medicine*, **343**, 1342–1343.

Rich S, Dantzker DR, Ayres SM, *et al.* (1987) Primary pulmonary hypertension. A national prospective study. *Annals of Internal Medicine*, **107**(2), 216–223.

Rubin LJ, Badesch DB & Barst RJ (2002) Bosentan therapy for pulmonary arterial hypertension *New England Journal of Medicine*, **346**, 896–903.

Wilkins H, Guth A, Konig J, *et al.* (2001) Effect of inhaled iloprost plus oral sildenafil in patients with primary pulmonary hypertension. *Circulation*, **104**, 1218–1222.

PART 3

Emergencies and Special Situations

CHAPTER 23

Arrhythmia and Syncope

Arrhythmia is part of the 'natural' history of many congenital heart lesions and their surgical repairs. Loss of sinus rhythm is one of the more common reasons for hospital admission. Unfortunately, in this group arrhythmias are often more difficult to detect (slow intra-atrial re-entry may superficially appear like sinus rhythm), associated with significant morbidity, resistant to drug therapy and challenging to treat in the electrophysiologic laboratory. In addition, palpitation alone can turn a young working adult into someone who is unable to hold down their job or function independently in the community.

Supraventricular rhythm disturbances are by far the most common arrhythmias to affect this group. In a compromised heart, a fast supraventricular rhythm can be as devastating as ventricular tachycardia. In particular, atrial flutter may be conducted 1:1 in this relatively young patient population and cause cardiovascular collapse. At the other end of the spectrum, it is essential that all high-risk subjects have regular 12-lead EKGs at their clinic visits to detect slow 'symptom-free' atrial flutter.

Rather than list the myriad arrhythmias that can be encountered in this population, we will focus on the practicalities of treating some of the most common rhythm upsets (see Table 23.1).

Atypical flutter (intra-atrial re-entry)

Atypical flutter or intra-atrial re-entry tachycardia (IART) is worth a special note. This is a common cause of palpitation in those with previous atrial surgery. Prior surgery and atrial stretch are the substrate for the development of multiple clockwise circuits around electrical barriers of suture lines and scarring. These palpitations recur frequently and often necessitate multiple admissions to hospital. Acutely, chemical cardioversion is rare and patients often need electrical cardioversion.

Beta-blockers and amiodarone are the most frequently used drug therapies. Other forms of preventive therapies such as atrial pacing and atrial defibrillators may reduce the number of acute episodes but rarely abolish the problem. Unlike traditional flutter, these flutter waves may be slow and inhomogeneous. Sometimes they are difficult to recognize, especially if the atrial rate is relatively slow. IART circuits are usually not isthmus-dependent and may need some of the newer mapping techniques to direct ablation.

Table 23.1

Rhythm	Common anatomy	Comments
Atypical atrial flutter (intra-atrial re-entry)	Mustard, Senning Fontan (esp. old style) Atrial septal defect (ASD) repairs	Often recur and require repeated electrical cardioversions Limited drug options if associated with impaired ventricular function Often multiple circuits when mapped in the EP lab (can exist alongside isthmus-dependent typical atrial flutter) Refractory flutter may be an indication for redo Fontan
Accessory pathway	Classically in Ebstein anomaly of the tricuspid valve	May terminate with intravenous adenosine in the emergency department Catheter ablation is the treatment of choice
Atrial fibrillation	ASD, esp. in elderly Poor systemic ventricular function	Can persist or develop despite ASD repair, esp. if over 40 years of age at the time of repair May represent other co-morbidity: hypertension, left ventricular dysfunction
Ventricular tachycardia	Myocardial disease Failing systemic ventricle Tetralogy of Fallot Ventricular septal defect: repaired	In tetralogy, a QRS duration of >180 ms is a risk factor Address and target residual hemodynamic lesions Need to consider if automated intracardiac defibrillator is appropriate Need to consider if ventricular tachycardia ablation is appropriate May present as sudden cardiac death

Ventricular tachycardia

Ventricular tachycardia (VT) is predominantly an issue for those with previous ventriculotomies (for ventricular septal defect and/or tetralogy repair from a different, earlier, surgical era), tetralogy subjects with severe pulmonary regurgitation and poor right ventricles and those with systemic ventricular dysfunction. This includes individuals with univentricular hearts, Fontans, and systemic right ventricles.

Risk stratification remains a challenge in this group, but a prolonged QRS duration has been shown to be a risk marker for sustained VT and sudden cardiac death, at least in the Fallot group. The significance of non-sustained VT (NSVT) on Holter or exercise is less clear. Identifying and addressing underlying target hemodynamic lesions in these patients is an integral part of arrhythmia management and risk modification. However, with or without redo surgery and arrhythmia targeting procedures, arrhythmia may recur longer term. Automated intracardiac defibrillators (AICDs) will, therefore, have an important role in these patients. Indications for AICD implantation, however, in this patient group are yet to be determined, but this is a potentially life-saving treatment option for many of these patients. Care must be taken in programming these devices, as congenital patients often also suffer from supraventricular arrhythmias. These patients need specialist care from an electrophysiologist with an understanding of congenital heart conditions.

Atrial arrhythmias and the atrial septal defect

Atrial flutter and fibrillation are commonly associated with atrial septal defects (ASDs). Early correction (under the age of 40 years) reduces the risk of palpitation but does not abolish it. Atrial wall stretch, right atrium fibrosis and pulmonary vein potentials are all arrhythmogenic substrates. In the short term, approximately two-thirds of patients with paroxysmal atrial flutter or fibrillation before ASD closure will improve following repair. However, arrhythmia is likely to return longer term, particularly in the older patient. Current best practice is to combine surgical closure with the MAZE procedure. In the setting of transcatheter closure, pulmonary vein ablation may become part of standard therapy. In this setting, it is important that these issues are addressed before closing the defect, and thus before interrupting the direct access to the left atrium for the electrophysiologist.

The congenital patient with an arrhythmia: emergency care

1 Assess hemodynamic compromise: institute basic resuscitation if needed. If unwell with hypotension, consider urgent electrical cardioversion.

2 Assess rhythm in the context of lesion, history and medication. A previous 12-lead resting sinus EKG is invaluable. A broad-complex tachycardia is often not VT in this setting. **Seek expert help early**. This may be a recurrent problem well known to the patient's congenital cardiologist.

3 Ascertain if anticoagulated and if effective (recent INRs).

4 High-risk patients should not remain in arrhythmia for anything but the minimum amount of time. Fontan patients and those with ventricular impairment need early cardioversion. A TOE may be needed to assess the presence of intracardiac clot if INRs have been <2.5 or if delayed presentation. (Beware of positive pressure ventilation in Fontan subjects having a detrimental effect on Fontan flow.)

5 Try to avoid anti-arrhythmics that are strongly negative inotropic in those with impaired hemodynamics. Avoid using multiple drugs. Assess prior QT intervals and try to avoid pro-arrhythmic medications.

6 In the setting of anti-arrhythmic drugs and electrical cardioversion, make plans for action if patient becomes bradycardic. Is transvenous pacing possible/necessary? Is there secure venous access, etc.?

7 **Seek expert help early**. If the patient is known to have recurrent refractory arrhythmia, for example, is 'acute' catheter ablation a possibility?

8 Consider prevention: anatomical substrate? Hemodynamic surgery? Drugs? Ablation? Devices?

9 Think very carefully before transferring a sick tachycardic patient to another unit. The patient is often best managed with phone/fax consultation, with transfer only taking place once stability is established.

Atypical atrial flutter (IART) in the emergency department

- Chemical cardioversion is *rarely successful.*
- Consider early (same day!) electrical cardioversion for all at-risk subjects.
- Amiodarone, intravenous beta-blockade and intravenous diltiazem are the most frequently used rate-control agents (while organizing cardioversion/anticoagulation).
- Remember the issue of anticoagulation.
- Low-threshold for TOE to exclude clot.

Prevention
Redo surgery
Typical example of a patient with an obstructed Fontan circuit and an 11 cm right atrium. No amount of drug therapy or any catheter intervention will guarantee restoration and maintenance of sinus rhythm. If surgery is being considered for a hemodynamic lesion in the context of palpitation, then specifically targeted electrophysiologic intervention (such as a surgical MAZE procedure) should be planned.

Why try to maintain sinus rhythm in these patients?

- Symptom control (optimizing hemodynamics).
- Improved effort capacity and exercise tolerance.
- Reduced thromboembolic risk (especially in Fontan subjects).
- Improve hemodynamics; patients may be dependent on atrial filling and AV synchrony (e.g. HOCM).
- Rate control is often poor in this young group.
- Reversion to SR is often easier to achieve early after onset.
- Possible survival benefits (e.g. Mustard group).

Drug therapy
Prescribing anti-arrhythmics can be difficult in this patient group. This is especially true for the sicker patients with poorer ventricular function. In addition, therapy may be needed for many decades, and therefore amiodarone's long-term side-effects may be particularly relevant, especially thyroid disorders. The effectiveness and adverse event profile of dofetalide is not yet established in this patient group.

Factors to consider when prescribing anti-arrhythmics

- Therapy may be needed lifelong.
- Patients are at increased risk of sinus and AV node pathology.
- Patients have conduction defects, prolonged QRS and QT intervals—beware pro-arrhythmic effects.
- Negative inotropes are poorly tolerated by single ventricles.
- Pregnancy may be an issue in female patients.
- In reality, the most commonly used drugs in this population are amiodarone and beta-blockers, including sotalol.

Ablation techniques

Ablation technologies continue to advance speedily. Improved mapping techniques (such as CARTO) and new catheters that can deliver deeper and more precise 'burns' are two developments that are especially useful in the congenital heart patient. These patients remain, however, challenging subjects with access problems, multiple circuits and thick atrial walls. Nevertheless, for many patients a successful ablation can have a major impact on quality of life and should be considered (in combination with hemodynamic intervention).

Pacing and devices

Pacing and devices have an increasing role in patients with congenital heart disease. They clearly need to be handled by an expert in the field. Access difficulties, residual shunts (risk of paradoxical embolism) and right atrium–pulmonary artery connections may be indications for epicardial pacing. Atrial defibrillators, ventricular defibrillators and biventricular pacing systems are all new modalities that are beginning to have a role and an impact on patient care. Relative indications, optimal timing and longer-term follow-up data need to be defined.

Syncope

Syncope is a concerning symptom in this patient group. This is especially true for the cyanotic patient or patient with pulmonary hypertension. Benign causes also occur in young adults, e.g. postural vasovasal syncope or early gestational syncope during pregnancy, but syncope should not be dismissed lightly.

Cardiovascular causes of syncope in congenital heart patients

- Tachyarrythmia (symptoms dependent on rate and hemodynamic substrate).
- Sinus node or AV node disease.
- Pulmonary thromboembolic disease.
- Impaired cardiac output due to obstructive lesions (e.g. conduit).
- Severe cyanosis.
- Acute prosthetic valve obstruction (thrombus).
- Dissection, aortic rupture.
- Ischemia.
- Drug-induced hypotension, especially postural.
- Simple vasovagal.
- Benign.

Patients require basic investigations to rule out anatomic or electrical abnormalities. These would include echocardiography, 12-lead EKG, and Holter monitoring. (Patient-activated recorders and loop recorders may also be needed.)

Note: in the setting of suspected PTE, there are many pitfalls in interpreting CT angiograms and ventilation:perfusion scans in these patients. This is especially true for those with shunts and systemic-to-pulmonary artery anastomoses.

It is good practice and should be encouraged that all patients with congenital heart disease have a copy of their resting sinus EKG in their personal records.

CHAPTER 24

Suspected Infective Endocarditis

Despite more sensitive diagnostic tests, the new generation of antibiotics and improved surgical techniques, endocarditis remains a potentially lethal disease. It is also a common cause of emergency admission for adults with congenital heart disease. Below is a clinical perspective rather than that of the microbiologist, epidemiologist or pathologist. For further information see Chapter 4.

Prevention

The prime focus for anyone caring for the congenital cardiac patient must remain prevention. This should be more than just ensuring that the patient knows to take antibiotics at the time of dental work.

The following education points are crucial:

1 An understanding of **why** antibiotics are prescribed prophylactically.
2 An understanding of **non-dental** procedures that may require prophylaxis.
3 Simple instructions about the basic care of **wounds** to prevent bacteremia.
4 Instructions about what to do in the event of a **febrile illness**.
5 In particular, patients should be encouraged to ask that **blood cultures** and bacteriology (urine, sputum, etc.) samples be taken before starting a course of blinded antibiotic therapy.
6 Patients should be informed of the **subacute** manifestations of endocarditis, e.g. unexplained weight loss and anorexia.

Endocarditis is a diagnosis that one would not want to miss. It should also be remembered that the majority of congenital cardiac patients with a temperature do not have infective endocarditis. However, the physician caring for large numbers of congenital patients will spend a reasonable amount of time excluding endocarditis in their patients (see below).

The congenital heart patient with a temperature

History
Key to diagnosis: with special reference to risk stratification
- History of predisposing event.
- Symptoms of hemodynamic decompensation.
- Systemic upset and symptoms of complications.

Examination
- Classic stigmata often absent.
- Careful examination of skin: rashes, entry points.

- New murmurs (requires previous description/documentation).
- Exclusion of other causes of fever.
- Hemodynamic upset: tachycardia, heart failure.

Blood work (minimum)
- Blood cultures.
- Full blood count with differential white cell count.
- Renal function.
- Liver function and proteins.
- Immunoglobulin, autoantibodies: if diagnosis unclear.
- C-reactive protein (serial).

Specimens
- Urine: urinalysis, culture and sensitivities (C&S).
- Sputum for C&S.
- Other microbiology specimens as appropriate.

Electrocardiogram
- Changes, especially new conduction defects.

Imaging
- Chest radiography: ? changes in CTR, parenchymal changes from embolic events.
- Echocardiography: initially transthoracic but low threshold for transesophageal imaging, especially if complex lesion is present (failure to detect vegetations does not exclude endocarditis).
- CT imaging/MR: for complications such as infective emboli and infarcts—brain, head, spleen.

Despite even the best of preventive care, endocarditis occurs. Often the source of infection remains unknown, with only about 40% of cases having an identifiable predisposing event (e.g. dental or cardiac surgery).

The commonest sites for endocarditis in the adult with a congenital heart lesion are a small ventricular septal defect, a stenotic left ventricular outflow tract or an obstructed right-sided conduit. The presence of any prosthetic cardiac material (patches, valves, conduits) is an added risk factor for infection. The most common pathogens continue to include streptococci, enterococci, staphylococci, and the HACEK organisms.

Diagnosis

The diagnosis of endocarditis has always been an area of difficulty. This is particularly true for those with congenital heart disease, especially if involving complex repairs or prosthetic intracardiac and intravascular material. In this group, the classic stigmata of endocarditis are often absent: evidence of active valvulitis, peripheral emboli and immunologic vascular phenomena. This is particularly true for acute endocarditis and right-sided lesions.

Most clinicians use the Duke diagnostic criteria, although these must be tailored with clinical experience of the congenital heart population (see Table 24.1). History, blood cultures and imaging remain the cornerstones of diagnosis.

Echocardiography

Even with modern imaging technology (predominantly echocardiography), the diagnosis of endocarditis is not simple and may be delayed. However, echocardiography remains an important diagnostic tool. Transthoracic echocardiography has a high specificity but low sensitivity for the detection of vegetations (<60%). Patients with complex congenital heart lesions, conduits, prosthetic valves and right-sided lesions are particularly difficult to image. In these groups there should be a low threshold for transesophageal imaging (TOE).

A negative TOE study does not exclude infective endocarditis and the patient's other diagnostic information should be reviewed thoroughly. In all comers, when both TTE and TOE are negative they have a 95% negative predictive value. The equivalent value for those with congenital lesions is unknown. However, if there is a persisting high clinical suspicion, repeat studies may be needed.

Echocardiography also has a role in monitoring response to treatment—be that vegetation size or hemodynamic sequelae. The complications of endocarditis may also be detected with careful imaging such as TOE assessment for aortic root abscess.

Table 24.1 Infective endocarditis (IE)

Pathological criteria
Microbiological and pathological evidence from a vegetation, or intracardiac abscess
Clinical criteria
2 major or 1 major and 3 minor or 5 minor
MAJOR criteria include:
Blood cultures: 2 separate positive blood cultures with a typical organism
Persistently positive cultures with an organism consistent with IE
Endocardial involvement
Positive echocardiogram with classic vegetation or abscess or new partial dehiscence of a prosthetic valve
New valvular regurgitation
MINOR criteria include:
Predisposition: heart condition or IVDA
Fever >38°C
Vascular phenomena
Immunologic phenomena
Microbiological evidence (not sufficient to be major)
Echocardiography finding (suggestive but not sufficient to be major)

Unusual organisms

The causes of culture-negative endocarditis are well recognized and more fully described in the ACC/AHA guidelines. Patients with cyanotic heart disease may have a degree of immunocompromise, and therefore unusual organisms (e.g. Q fever or fungal infections) may be more common.

Other pointers towards fungal endocarditis include the presence of large vegetations, metastatic infection and perivalvular invasion. The prognosis in this group is poor.

Treatment

Good communication with the microbiologist or infectious diseases specialist remains key to effective treatment of infective endocarditis. Prolonged antibiotic therapy and intravenous access may be problematic in congenital heart patients who have had multiple previous lines and procedures. Peripherally placed intravenous central catheters (PICC) may be a less traumatic option than Hickman or other central lines.

Surgery

It is always wise to inform the congenital cardiac surgical team if a congenital patient develops endocarditis (even if this surgeon is at the regional center). Early discussion and planning for the eventualities of treatment failure or complications may optimize care should things not settle with medical therapy. Below are documented key failures that act as 'surgical alarm bells'.

Although cardiac surgery may be undertaken in an urgent setting, it is imperative that whenever possible surgery is performed by an experienced congenital cardiac surgeon. Perioperative mortality for these patients remains high.

Possible indications for consideration of surgical intervention

- A pre-existing indication for surgery.
- Enlarging vegetations despite appropriate antibiotic therapy.
- Embolic events despite antibiotic therapy.
- Worsening valvular disease: increasing regurgitation.
- Valve leaflet rupture/perforation.
- Heart failure.
- Perivalvular extension, e.g. aortic root abscess, new conduction defects.
- *Staphylococcus aureus* infection, especially in the presence of prosthetic material.

Key clinical points

- A low index of suspicion in high-risk patients, especially if previous infective endocarditis.
- Beware of *Staphylococcus aureus* endocarditis: this is a virulent and aggressive organism in the setting of prosthetic material.

• Beware of aortic valve endocarditis: patients should have their cardiac rhythm monitored; heart block suggests root abscess; communicate with the surgeons.

• Beware the patient with aortic endocarditis and severe aortic regurgitation. Beware low diastolic pressures (coronary ischemia) and rapid onset of left ventricular and renal failure.

• Don't forget the possibility of central nervous system involvement: if new neurologic signs, reduction in level of consciousness or changes in behavior develop, consider mycotic aneurysms and cerebral abscess.

CHAPTER 25

Perioperative Care

It is common for the adult with congenital heart disease to require non-cardiac surgery, for example, a dental or obstetric procedure. The majority of patients, even if treated surgically in early life, will have important residual or associated lesions that may affect their perioperative outcome.

The key to managing patients with congenital heart disease is anticipation and elimination of problems and recruitment of appropriate specialist knowledge beforehand. There are no formal studies documenting risk stratification in congenital heart patients undergoing non-cardiac surgery, but it is possible to identify those who may run into difficulties.

If patients have moderate or complex congenital heart disease, complex surgery is contemplated, or there are adverse risk factors (including poor functional class, pulmonary hypertension, CHF and cyanosis) the assessment and the surgery should be performed in a regional adult congenital heart disease center.

Preoperative risk stratification

Cardiac factors
- Residual systemic-to-pulmonary shunts.
- Residual right-to-left shunts: risk of paradoxical embolism.
- Cyanosis (with associated complications, e.g. renal, hematological).
- Pulmonary hypertension.
- Poor ventricular function.
- Arrhythmias.
- Prosthetic valves: function especially obstructive, anticoagulation.
- Fontan circulation.

Presence of co-morbidity
- Hypertension, diabetes, renal dysfunction.
- Bleeding disorders, e.g. in cyanosed patients.
- Lung disease (e.g. restrictive physiology due to scoliosis).

Surgical issues
- High-risk procedures, e.g. excess bleeding, metabolic upset.

Outline of perioperative management

Low-risk lesions
• Written perioperative instructions from a cardiologist with a special interest in congenital heart disease: may help to minimize excessive concern and over-management (*minimum requirement*).

High-risk lesions
• Perioperative planning with cardiac anesthetist, surgeon and congenital specialist.

Specific consideration of:
• where surgery should be performed;
• where postoperative care should take place;
• invasive monitoring required;
• specialist input required;
• special equipment required: e.g. nitric oxide, pacing, etc.

The congenital cardiologist should clarify the diagnosis, the physiology, residual sequelae and management strategies. An experienced cardiac anesthetist should advise regarding access, monitoring and ventilation issues.

Such documents serve as invaluable references for those directly involved in the 24-hour care of the patient perioperatively.

The patient should be in the best possible health for elective procedures:

• Optimize the treatment of heart failure.
• Treat hypertension.
• Consider treating significant obstructive lesions before elective procedures.
• Consider beta-blockade for perioperative ischemic and arrhythmic risk.
• Check thyroid function (Down syndrome; those on amiodarone).
• Consider autologous blood donation.
• Consider withholding diuretics and vasodilators on the day of surgery.

Issues that require special preoperative consideration

Anticoagulation
Anticoagulation is an important cause of perioperative morbidity and extended hospital stay. Special care should be taken in those with non-sinus rhythm, previous thrombotic events, mitral valve replacements and a Fontan circulation.

Cyanosis
Cyanosis is associated with an increased risk of bleeding (abnormal platelet function and coagulation factors, increased tissue vascularity, and collaterals). Preoperative isovolumic phlebotomy may improve hemostatic function (increases

platelet levels). Dehydration should be avoided, as this may precipitate symptoms of hyperviscosity. Anticoagulation carries a significant risk in this group, compounded by the fact that laboratory error is common in prothrombin time (PT) and activated partial thromboplastin time (APTT) measurements in this group.

Pulmonary hypertension
The presence of severe pulmonary hypertension turns even the most minor procedure into one associated with considerable risk. There is little capacity to increase pulmonary blood flow and the cardiac output is relatively fixed. There is a trade-off between increasing cardiac output and increasing shunting (exacerbating cyanosis).

Ventricular dysfunction
The risk is in proportion to the degree of ventricular dysfunction. This is true for the systemic left ventricle, right ventricle or single ventricle. Treatment of heart failure should be optimized before surgery, whereas negative inotropic drugs should be avoided.

Ventricular outflow tract obstruction
Fluid overload of these patients may provoke pulmonary edema or right heart failure. Hypovolemia will also be poorly tolerated by further compromising cardiac output.

Rhythm abnormalities
Arrhythmias may occur for numerous reasons including the cardiac condition per se, worsening of hemodynamics, drug therapies, metabolic upset and lung disease. Patients with atrioventricular block may need perioperative pacing. This could be planned electively with special consideration given to the forms of pacing possible and the available access, e.g. in Fontan patients. Patients with pacemakers or defibrillators should have their device assessed preoperatively. Defibrillators may be activated by cautery.

Endocarditis prophylaxis
When bacteremia is anticipated.

Anesthetic technique

Choice of specific anesthetic agents
Drugs such as narcotics and low-dose inhalational agents cause less upset to the systemic vascular bed. Vasodilators, diuretic and nitric oxide may all be needed in the early postoperative period.

Do not assume that local anesthetic techniques are 'safer' (for example, spinal anesthesia may lower systemic vascular resistance (SVR) and cause hypotension). Epidural anesthesia is preferred, as dosing can be tailored to the patient.

Vascular access

Planning: anatomy, the needs of the surgeon, previous access difficulties should be taken into consideration.

Air embolism and paradoxical embolism: bubble traps are not effective when administering viscous drugs, e.g. propofol or blood products.

In the planning of a surgical procedure and the postoperative care, intra-operative monitoring must be tailored to the patient's cardiac condition and to the surgical procedure.

• Non-invasive blood pressure monitoring: remember that those with a BT shunt or coarctation repair may have asymmetrical or absent pulses.
• Transcutaneous or intra-arterial oxygen saturation.
• Pulse monitoring (especially if paced).
• Intra-arterial blood pressure monitoring: beat to beat assessment is important when changes in circulating fluid volumes or vascular resistance are expected.
• Pulmonary artery pressure monitoring is especially hazardous in this patient group (e.g. in those with pulmonary hypertension and intra-atrial shunts) and should be undertaken only when the benefits outweigh these risks. Remember the anatomy of the Glenn and Fontan patients!
• Intra-operative transesophageal echocardiography for ventricular function: performed by an operator with congenital echo expertise.

Fontan circulation

The patient with a Fontan circulation warrants specific mention.

Desaturation

Patients with a Fontan procedure should have essentially normal saturations unless associated with large fenestrations, 'anomalous' coronary sinus drainage, venous–venous collateral vessels draining into the systemic atrium or arteriovenous malformations in the lung.

Pulmonary blood flow

Lung blood flow is dependent on adequate filling pressures and pulmonary resistance. Any factor affecting pulmonary pressures may impair cardiac output (postoperative atelectasis, pulmonary embolism or pneumothorax). Many factors may reduce the preload such as hemorrhage, vasodilators, over-diuresis and increases in intrathoracic pressure such as positive pressure ventilation. Such changes may be catastrophic for the Fontan patient.

Vascular access

Anatomy should be remembered, especially if considering urgent transvenous pacing or pulmonary artery pressure monitoring!

Specific postoperative issues

When high-risk cardiac patients or high-risk surgical procedures are involved, patients are best managed in an acute care area such as the intensive care unit or coronary care unit. Complications (bleeding, infection, fever, thrombosis, embolism, fluid overload, dehydration) need to be detected early and treated aggressively. Optimizing postoperative pain control will help reduce catecholamine stress. Early discharge is inadvisable.

Emergency surgery in the non-specialist unit

If the patient presents acutely with a surgical emergency, there may not be time for a full preoperative evaluation. The patient or their family being fully aware and able to provide relevant information and documentation of the patient's cardiac diagnosis is invaluable. Complex patients may also consider the use of a Medicare bracelet. In addition, expert help should be sought at the earliest point, and definitely in the postoperative period.

CHAPTER 26

Heart Failure: Acute Management

In treating patients who present acutely it is imperative that there is an under-standing of their cardiac anatomy and physiology. Attempting, for example, to diurese a Fontan subject on the basis of their JVP (which should be elevated, reflecting the atrial-to-pulmonary artery communication) can have devastat-ing consequences. Many of these patients have very finely balanced hemody-namics and over-aggressive use of vasodilators may be dangerous.

The acute presentation with classic 'left heart' (systemic heart) failure with pulmonary edema is relatively uncommon in this patient group. In general, chronic poor systemic cardiac output and right heart (subpulmonary) failure are more frequent problems.

In any patient with an acute onset of ventricular dysfunction, an underlying cause needs to be excluded. This most commonly will be arrhythmic. In addi-tion, a new anatomical substrate, underlying infection or ischemic event should be considered.

Lesions that may present with 'systemic heart failure' symptoms

- Mitral valve disease (mitral stenosis may mimic systolic ventricular failure).
- Acute severe aortic regurgitation.
- Aortic stenosis (rarely an acute presentation in the young).
- Unrepaired coarctation with ventricular dysfunction (rare).
- Mustard patients with systemic right ventricular (RV) failure.
- CCTGA with systemic RV failure.
- Systemic left ventricular (LV) dysfunction, e.g. elderly tetralogy patient.
- Pulmonary vein obstruction; may mimic pulmonary edema: rare.
- Myocardial disease, e.g. DMD.

Right heart (subpulmonary) heart failure is a more common problem. This, how-ever, usually presents subacutely in keeping with anatomic and functional decline. Symptoms may progress insidiously with abdominal distension, anorexia, weight loss and deranged liver function, pain, as well as frank edema and ascites. Cachexia is a worrying symptom and may increase perioperative morbidity and even mortal-ity (if heart failure data from purely ischemic heart disease can be extrapolated).

Lesions that may present with 'right heart failure' symptoms

- Fontan (raised right atrial pressure, arrhythmia, protein-losing enteropathy).
- Pulmonary hypertension (multiple causes).
- Large atrial septal defects (especially in the elderly).

- Tricuspid valve disease (stenosis or regurgitation, but rare in Ebstein).
- Right ventricle–pulmonary artery conduit stenosis (e.g. Rastelli).
- Mustard with baffle obstruction.
- Severe pulmonary regurgitation with RV dilatation.
- (Don't forget new or chronic pulmonary thromboembolic disease.)

Treatment of left- and right-sided failure

Treatment should be directed to the underlying causes. Diuretics clearly will not cure a severely stenosed conduit! The first rule of drug therapy is to first 'do no wrong'. Drug therapy should be used with caution but can be highly effective. There is, unfortunately, little to no evidence base for the use of many of the standard heart failure drugs in this population. However, a few recent studies suggest that similar mechanisms may be involved. There is evidence, for example, of neurohormonal activation in many of these patients.

Specific caution in this population is required because of the increased incidence of renal impairment. This may limit drug availability, effectiveness and overall outcome.

In the setting of palliative care of end-stage heart disease, control of symptoms is key. In this setting, use of inotropes and placement of central lines does little to alter outcome and may be inappropriate.

Device therapy
There is little data on the use of intra-aortic balloon pumping outwith the perioperative period. However, mechanical assistance, whether balloon pumping or assist devices, may be an important adjunct in this patient group. This is especially true if there is an expected degree of reversibility to the decline.

The Fontan patient
Patients presenting with edema in the setting of a Fontan are a particular problem and require specialist treatment (see Table 26.1). Protein-losing enteropathy with resistant edema has a grave prognosis. In addition, non-sinus rhythm and Fontan obstruction need to be excluded.

Heart failure drugs in congenital heart disease

The patient presenting with 'failure'

1 Basic ABC of resuscitation if appropriate.
2 What is the anatomy and what does that mean?
3 Is there a new acute hemodynamic lesion that needs urgent intervention (e.g. a ruptured mitral valve chordea)?
4 Is the patient in sinus rhythm? If not, consider cardioversion.
5 Is there evidence of infective endocarditis or systemic infection?
6 Does the patient have a Fontan repair?

Table 26.1 Drug therapy for heart failure in patients with congenital heart disease

	Advantages	Disadvantages
Loop diuretics	Highly effective in symptom control	Caution if pre-load-dependent Caution with renal function Absorption may be impaired in chronically edematous patients
Spironolactone	Effective for right-sided failure symptom control	Mortality benefits in this group?
ACEI (and to a lesser extent angiotensin-2 inhibitors)	Used in the treatment of hypertension and ventricular failure in this group	Mortality benefits in this group? Little evidence to support use Beware if pre-load-dependent Beware renal function Beware if obstructive lesions present
Beta-blockers	Anti-arrhythmic Good for HR control, e.g. mitral stenosis	Mortality benefits in this group? Caution regarding conduction defects
Digoxin	Rate control of permanent AF Parallel therapy to other anti-arrhythmic drugs	Often overprescribed in this group Benefits in this group re. failure?
Nitrates		Rarely used clinically in this group Patients often borderline hypotensive
Opiates	May be useful in palliative care of end-stage/terminal heart failure	

7 What is the site of the problem: LV? RV? both?

8 What is the main problem: poor cardiac output, peripheral edema, pulmonary edema?

9 What are the disadvantages of giving drug A on systemic output, filling pressures, kidneys, etc.?

10 Where will this line end up if I attempt to gain access (especially true for patients with Fontan and Glenn repairs and left-sided superior vena cavas)?

It should be emphasized that these patients are difficult to manage when acutely unwell. Classic signs of raised JVPs, basal crepitations and edema may be obscured by their longstanding pathologies. *Expert advice should be sought as soon as possible.*

CHAPTER 27

Care of the Cyanosed Patient

This chapter is an overview of the care of this very special group of patients with a variety of conditions. For more information about specific lesions and their most appropriate therapy, please see the lesion-specific chapters and the chapter on pulmonary hypertension and on Eisenmenger complex.

Cyanosis (a blue discoloration of the skin) is caused by an increased amount of reduced hemoglobin (non-oxygenated). In congenital cardiac patients, this is usually a manifestation of either:

1 *mixing of oxygenated and non-oxygenated blood*
   • right-to-left shunting
   • univentricular heart
or
2 *inadequate pulmonary blood flow*
   • underdeveloped pulmonary vasculature
   • progressive pulmonary hypertension.

Therefore, a variety of cardiac lesions may be associated with cyanosis, and cyanosis is not synonymous with an Eisenmenger reaction. For example, a very large atrial septal defect may be associated with cyanosis secondary to mixing of right atrial and left atrial blood rather than irreversible pulmonary hypertension and reverse shunting.

The commoner causes of cyanosis in the adult

Simple shunts with Eisenmenger physiology
• Ventricular septal defect
• Atrial septal defect (rare in secundum)
• Patent ductus arteriosus
• Aortopulmonary window

Complex lesions without Eisenmenger physiology
• Transposition of the great arteries*
• Truncus arteriosus*
• Tetralogy of Fallot/pulmonary stenosis with ventricular septal defect*
• Tetralogy of Fallot with pulmonary atresia*
• Univentricular heart*
• Tricuspid atresia
• Ebstein's anomaly with atrial septal defect

- Complete atrioventricular canal defect*
- Previous classic Glen shunt with pulmonary arteriovenous malformations

*May have pulmonary hypertension also.

The presence of a reduced oxygen level sets into motion a variety of secondary compensatory mechanisms. These include the following.

1 Attempts to increase oxygen content.
2 An increase in hemoglobin.
3 A rightwards shift in the oxygen dissociation curve.
4 Increased cardiac output.

The multi-organ impact of cyanotic heart diseases

There are many adaptive and pathologic changes associated with chronic cyanosis and it is often difficult to separate the adaptive from the 'maladaptive'. Chapter 20 fully documents the secondary consequences of chronic cyanosis.

Treatment

Treatment of the cyanosed patient is highly dependent on the underlying cardiac lesion and its 'reparability'. In those with no further surgical, transcatheter or transplant options, limited measures may palliate symptoms.

Oxygen therapy

Nocturnal oxygen may be helpful in improving wellbeing in some patients. In addition, as-required oxygen administration may also improve symptoms.

Venesection

In the past, venesection has been inappropriately used in an attempt to normalize hemoglobin levels. This was done to reduce a perceived risk of thrombosis. This is no longer standard practice. Venesection should only be performed for:

1 convincing hyperviscosity symptoms (in the absence of dehydration or severe iron deficiency);
2 preoperatively for hematocrit >65% (especially if thrombocytopenia is an issue).

Venesection should only be performed 1 unit at a time and the volume withdrawn should be replaced by normal saline in a controlled manner.

Iron deficiency should be treated with pulses of low-dose iron replacement to avoid excessive rebound.

Hemoglobin levels per se should not be used as an indication for venesection. In general, the hemoglobin will be inversely proportional to the oxygen saturation level of the patient.

Patient education

It is important that the patient be aware of his or her own resting oxygen levels when well. This should hopefully minimize the risks of unnecessary oxygen administration, over-investigation or inappropriate intubation.

Pregnancy

The maternal risk associated with cyanosis and pregnancy varies depending on the etiology of the cyanosis. A patient with pulmonary atresia and a shunt is more likely to tolerate pregnancy than a cyanotic patient with pulmonary vascular disease. Pregnancy in the Eisenmenger patient carries up to 50% mortality. Moreover, cyanosis (<85%) is still a significant risk factor for adverse neonatal outcomes. Pregnancy, therefore, should be discouraged prior to full assessment of the patient followed by discussion of the maternal and neonatal risks involved.

Cyanosis is poorly tolerated by the fetus. Miscarriage, prematurity and low birth weight are all common and proportional to the degree of cyanosis. Prolonged bed rest and oxygen therapy have anecdotally increased fetal growth and improved neonatal outcome, but this may not always be fruitful.

Role of anticoagulants

There is little or no role for anticoagulants or antiplatelets in those with cyanosis per se. However, in those with Eisenmenger physiology/pulmonary hypertension anticoagulants may have a role in the prevention of in situ thrombosis.

In patients treated with anticoagulants for another indication (e.g. atrial fibrillation or metallic valve), control of the INR can be challenging. The presence of extreme erythrocytosis can interfere with the laboratory assessment of INR. *It is important to involve the local hematology team in the management of these patients.*

Common clinical complications

- Bleeding secondary to low platelet levels and impaired clotting factors
- Infections, especially chest
- Hemoptysis (especially if pulmonary vascular disease)
- Pulmonary in situ thrombosis (especially if pulmonary vascular disease)
- Iron deficiency (exacerbated by venesection)
- Renal dysfunction

Paradoxical embolism

Those with intracardiac shunts are at risk of paradoxical embolism. This is particularly important in the context of transvenous pacing and the use of intravenous lines. Bubble traps should be used in those at risk.

Intervention options

Intervention options include percutaneous closure of intracardiac shunts, palliative surgical interventions to alter pulmonary blood flow or physiologic repair.

Systemic arterial-to-pulmonary artery shunts are used to improve pulmonary blood flow. Their long-term complications, however, include pulmonary hypertension from excessive pulmonary blood flow, pulmonary artery distortion and volume overload of the systemic ventricle. The role of late palliative shunts in adults is less clear.

There are also numerous catheter procedures that may improve pulmonary blood flow, for example, dilating or stenting old shunts or major aortopulmonary collateral arteries (MAPCAs). These are often difficult procedures to plan and execute and should be attempted only after multidisciplinary discussion. Their value in the adult is probably limited.

Transplantation of heart, one or both lungs with surgical repair or heart–lung transplantation have been performed in cyanotic patients. Pulmonary vascular obstructive disease precludes isolated heart transplantation.

Particular groups who do badly at transplantation include those with pulmonary atresia and MAPCAs due to excessive bleeding and those with multiple thoracotomies.

Key points

• Cyanosis is not equal to Eisenmenger's and may be due to variable cardiac morphology and physiology.
• Cyanosed patients have delicately balanced hemodynamics and should be cared for by specialists in congenital heart disease.

Bibliography

Diagnosis and Management of Adult Congenital Heart Disease by **Michael A. Gatzoulis, Gary D. Webb, Piers Daubeney. Churchill Livingstone; 2003**
This practical resource provides essential guidance on the anatomic issues, clinical presentation, diagnosis and clinical management of adults with congenital heart disease. Each consistently structured, disease-oriented chapter discusses incidence, genetics, morphology, presentation, investigation and imaging, treatment and intervention. A wealth of illustrations, including line drawings, EKGs, radiographs and echocardiograms clearly depict the clinical manifestations of congenital defects.

Congenital Heart Disease in Adults by **Joseph K. Perloff, John S. Child. W B Saunders; 2nd edition 1998**
Clinical reference for cardiologists. Perloff and Child's book provides excellent clinical information on the special needs and concerns faced in caring for adults with congenital heart disease. First textbook of its kind in the field.

Congenital Heart Disease Adult by **Welton M. Gersony, Marlon, S. Rosenbaum, Myron L. Weisfeldt. McGraw-Hill Professional; 2001**
This guide to the broad spectrum of congenital heart defects helps to optimize adult patient care.

Congenital Heart Disease in Adults: A Practical Guide by **Andrew Redington, Darryl Shore, Paul Oldershaw. W B Saunders; 1997**
Concise text for cardiologists and family practitioners on the special aspects of managing congenital heart disease in adults. Takes the approach that these adults can't be treated as large children with congenital disease.

Cardiac Surgery by **Nicholas Kouchoukos, Eugene Blackstone, Donald Doty, Frank Hanley, Robert Karp. W B Saunders; 3rd edition 2003**
Essential textbook in both adult and pediatric cardiac surgery, updated and revised in a new, third edition. It thoroughly covers the full range of new and classic surgical procedures and presents the up-to-date clinical evidence specialists need to make effective management decisions.

Moss and Adams' Heart Disease in Infants, Children, and Adolescents: Including the Fetus and Young Adult **by Hugh D. Allen, Howard P. Gutgesell, Edward B. Clark, David J. Driscoll. Lippincott Williams & Wilkins; 6th edition 2000**
Updated throughout, the sixth edition of Moss and Adams continues to be the primary cardiology text for those who care for infants, children, adolescents, young adults, and fetuses with heart disease. A comprehensive text covering basic science theory through clinical practice of cardiovascular disease in the young, this edition includes an expanded special section on young adults and a greatly expanded genetics section.

Color Atlas of Congenital Heart Disease: Morphologic and Clinical Correlation **by Sew Yen Ho, E.J. Baker, M.L. Rigby, R.H. Anderson. Mosby; 1994**
A correlation of the clinical and pathological features of congenital heart disease, including anatomy, imaging and pathology. This work covers all aspects of structural defects of the heart and major vessels arising during the development of the fetus, as well as conditions seen in neonates and young children. It provides a comprehensive review of incidence and actuality of various conditions, their characteristic features as defined by a range of investigative techniques, and detailed discussion of underlying pathology.

Paediatric Cardiology **by Robert Anderson, E. Baker, M. Rigby, E. Shinebourne, M. Tynan. Churchill Livingstone; 2nd edition 2003**
A comprehensive and exhaustive reference of fundamental and clinical aspects of heart disease in infancy and childhood. The contributors are well-known experts in the field and the editors are a world-class group who have published extensively in the field. Provides an up-to-date and authoritative account of pediatric cardiovascular fields covering embryology, morphology, pathophysiology, specific clinical conditions, treatments and the psychosocial aspects of caring for patients with heart disease.

Cardiac Arrhythmias after Surgery for Congenital Heart Disease **by S. Balaji, P.C. Gillette, C.L. Case. Hodder Arnold; 2001**
This comprehensive text discusses all aspects of atrial and ventricular cardiac arrhythmias in patients undergoing cardiac surgery for congenital heart problems. This area is one of growing interest, as an increasing number of individuals with heart defects live longer due to improved therapy, and are now facing new problems. The numbers and types of problems being tackled by invasive ablation techniques have been growing dramatically since the mid-1980s, and this publication aims to tie together the aspects of these conditions. Appropriate management of these patients critically depends on knowledge of the type of surgery, the types of arrhythmias these patients are prone to, and the therapeutic modalities that can be used to treat them.

'Congenital Heart Disease in Adults' by Judith Therrien and Gary D. Webb. In *Heart Disease: A Textbook of Cardiovascular Medicine*, 6th edition. Edited by Eugene Braunwald, Douglas P. Zipes, Peter Libby. Saunders; 2001
The essential *Textbook of Cardiovascular Medicine*, bringing cutting-edge advances in the field. Ninety-eight world authorities synthesize everything from the newest findings in molecular biology and genetics to the latest imaging modalities, interventional procedures and medications. The two adult congenital heart editors Drs Therrien and Webb in this latest edition encompass all of today's essential knowledge in the field.

Task Force on the Management of Cardiovascular Diseases During Pregnancy of the European Society of Cardiology
Expert consensus document on management of cardiovascular diseases during pregnancy. *European Heart Journal*, 2003, **24**, 761–781.

Canadian Cardiovascular Society Consensus Conference 2001 update
Can J Cardiol **2001** Sep; **17:** 940–59; *Can J Cardiol* **2001** Oct; **17:** 1029–50; *Can J Cardiol* **2001** Nov; **17:** 1135–58

Task Force on the Management of Grown Up Congenital Heart Disease of the European Society of Cardiology
Eur Heart J **2003, 24,** 1035–84.

Glossary

Prepared for the CCS Consensus Conference 2001 update: Recommendations for the Management of Adults with Congenital Heart Disease, published in *Canadian Journal of Cardiology* 2001; 17(9); 943ff. and accessible online at: http://www.ccs.ca/society/conferences/archives/2001/glossary.cfm and http://www.achd-library.com

Prepared by Jack M. Colman MD, FRCPC, FACC, Erwin Oechslin MD, FESC, and Dylan Taylor MD, FRCPC, FACC.

From *The ACHD Textbook: Diagnosis and Management of Adult Congenital Heart Disease* (eds MA Gatzoulis, GD Webb & P Daubeney) Philadelphia, PA: Churchill Livingstone, 2003.
Correspondence:
Jack M. Colman MD
Toronto Congenital Cardiac Centre for Adults
at the Toronto General Hospital/UHN
1603–600 University Avenue
Toronto ON M5G 1X5

The purpose of this glossary is to help guide those reading and researching in the area of adult congenital heart disease. It is meant to be a living document, constantly under revision, improvement, correction, as you, its users, find ways to ease the path for those who follow. To this end, if you cannot find a term you think should be here, or if you disagree with a definition, or see a way to improve it, drop us an e-mail before you move on. We promise to consider all feedback carefully, and to make additions and revisions on the website (http://www.achd-library.com/) often. We hope you find the glossary helpful.
Jack Colman: j.colman@utoronto.ca
Erwin Oechslin: erwin.oechslin@usz.ch
Dylan Taylor: dtaylor@cha.ab.ca

Acknowledgment: we recognize with gratitude the ongoing contribution of Dr Robert Freedom, who generously agreed to review the work. We appreciate his support and encouragement.

aberrant innominate artery
A rare abnormality associated with right aortic arch wherein the sequence of arteries arising from the aortic arch is: right carotid artery, right subclavian artery, then (left) innominate artery. The latter passes behind the esophagus. This is in contrast to the general rule that the first arch artery gives rise to the carotid artery contralateral to the side of the aortic arch (i.e. right carotid artery in left aortic arch and left carotid artery in right aortic arch). *syn.* retro-esophageal innominate artery.

aberrant subclavian artery
The right subclavian artery arises from the aorta distal to the left subclavian artery. Left aortic arch with (retroesophageal) aberrant right subclavian artery is the most common aortic arch anomaly, first described in 1735 by Hunauld, and occurring in 0.5% of the general population.

absent pulmonary valve syndrome
Pulmonary valvular tissue is absent, resulting in pulmonary regurgitation. This rare anomaly uncommonly may be isolated; or it may be associated with ventricular septal defect, obstructed pulmonary valve annulus and massive dilatation and distortion of the pulmonary arteries. Absent pulmonary valve may also occur in association with other simple or complex congenital heart lesions.

ACHD
Adult congenital heart disease.

Alagille syndrome
see arteriohepatic dysplasia.

ALCAPA
Anomalous left coronary artery arising from the pulmonary artery. *see* Bland-White-Garland syndrome.

ambiguus
With reference to cardiac situs, neither right- nor left-sided (indeterminate). *see* situs.

Amplatzer® device
A self-centering device delivered percutaneously by catheter for closure of an atrial septal defect, a patent foramen ovale or a patent ductus arteriosus.

anomalous pulmonary venous connection
Pulmonary venous return to the right heart, which may be total or partial.
• total anomalous pulmonary venous connection (TAPVC). All pulmonary veins connect to the right side of the heart, either directly or via venous tributaries. The connection may be supradiaphragmatic, usually via a vertical vein

to the innominate vein or the superior vena cava (SVC). The connection may also be infradiaphragmatic via a descending vein to the portal vein, the inferior vena cava (IVC) or one of its tributaries. Pulmonary venous obstruction is common in supradiaphragmatic connection, and almost universal in infradiaphragmatic connection.

• partial anomalous pulmonary venous connection (PAPVC). One or more but not all the pulmonary veins connect to the right atrium directly, or via a vena cava. This anomaly is frequently associated with sinus venosus atrial septal defect. *see also* scimitar syndrome.

aortic arch anomalies
Abnormalities of the aortic arch and its branching. Note that left or right aortic arch is defined by the mainstem bronchus that is crossed by the descending thoracic aorta and does not refer to the side of the midline on which the aorta descends.

In left aortic arch (normal anatomic arrangement) the descending thoracic aorta crosses over the left mainstem bronchus; the innominate artery branching into the right carotid and right subclavian artery arises first, the left carotid artery second and the left subclavian artery third. Usually, the first aortic arch vessel gives rise to the carotid artery that is opposite to the side of the aortic arch (i.e. the right carotid artery in left aortic arch and the left carotid artery in right aortic arch).The most important anomalies are:

• *abnormal left aortic arch*
  – left aortic arch with minor branching anomalies;
  – left aortic arch with retroesophageal right subclavian artery.
• *right aortic arch*. In right aortic arch the descending thoracic aorta crosses the right mainstem bronchus. It is often associated with tetralogy of Fallot, pulmonary atresia, truncus arteriosus and other cono-truncal anomalies. Types of right aortic arch branching include:
  – mirror image branching (left innominate artery, right carotid artery, right subclavian artery);
  – retroesophageal left (aberrant) subclavian artery with a normal calibre. Sequence of branching: left carotid artery, right carotid artery, right subclavian artery, then left subclavian artery;
  – retroesophageal diverticulum of Kommerell. *see* diverticulum of Kommerell;
  – right aortic arch with left descending aorta, i.e. retroesophageal segment of right aortic arch. The descending aortic arch crosses the midline toward the left by a retroesophageal route;
  – isolation of contralateral arch vessels: an aortic arch vessel arises from the pulmonary artery via the ductus arteriosus without connection to the aorta. This anomaly is very uncommon. Isolation of the left subclavian artery is the most common form.
• *cervical aortic arch*. The arch is located above the level of the clavicle.
• *double aortic arch*. Both right and left aortic arches are present, i.e. the ascending aorta splits into two limbs encircling the trachea and esophagus. The two

limbs join to form a single descending aorta. There are several forms such as widely open right and left arches or hypoplasia/atresia of one arch (usually the left). This anomaly is commonly associated with patent ductus arteriosus. Double aortic arch creates a vascular ring around the trachea and the esophagus. *see also* vascular ring.

• *persistent 5th aortic arch.* Double-lumen aortic arch with both lumina on the same side of the trachea. Degree of lumen patency varies from full patency of both lumina to complete atresia of one of them. Seen in some patients with coarctation of the aorta or interruption of the aortic arch.

• *interrupted aortic arch.* Complete discontinuation between the ascending and descending thoracic aorta.

   – Type A: interruption distal to the subclavian artery that is ipsilateral to the second carotid artery.

   – Type B: interruption between second carotid artery and ipsilateral subclavian artery.

   – Interruption between carotid arteries.

aortic-left ventricular defect (tunnel)
Vascular connection between the aorta and the left ventricle resulting in left ventricular volume overload due to regurgitation from the aorta via the tunnel to the left ventricle.

aortic override
see tetralogy of Fallot.

aortic valve-sparing ascending aortic replacement
see David operation.

aorto-pulmonary collateral
Abnormal arterial vessel arising from the aorta, providing blood supply to the pulmonary arteries. May be single or multiple, and small or large (see also MAPCA). May be associated with tetralogy of Fallot, pulmonary atresia or other complex cyanotic congenital heart disease.

aorto-pulmonary septal defect
see aorto-pulmonary window.

aorto-pulmonary window
A congenital connection between the ascending aorta and main pulmonary artery, which may be contiguous with the semi-lunar valves, or, less often, separated from them. Simulates the physiology of a large PDA, but requires a more demanding repair. *syn.* aorto-pulmonary septal defect.

arterial switch operation
see Jatene procedure.

arteriohepatic dysplasia

An autosomal dominant multisystem syndrome consisting of intrahepatic cholestasis, characteristic facies, butterfly-like vertebral anomalies and varying degrees of peripheral pulmonary artery stenoses or diffuse hypoplasia of the pulmonary artery and its branches. Associated with microdeletion in chromosome 20p. *syn.* Alagille syndrome.

asplenia syndrome

see isomerism/right isomerism.

atresia, atretic

Imperforate, used with reference to an orifice, valve, or vessel.

atrial septal defect (ASD)

an inter-atrial communication, classified according to its location relative to the oval fossa (fossa ovalis):

• coronary sinus ASD. Inferior and anterior location at the anticipated site of the orifice of the coronary sinus. May be part of a complex anomaly including absence of the coronary sinus and a persistent left superior vena cava.

• ostium primum ASD. Part of the spectrum of atrioventricular septal defect (AVSD). Located anterior and inferior to the oval fossa such that there is no atrial septal tissue between the lower edge of the defect and the atrioventricular valves that are located on the same plane; almost always associated with a 'cleft' in the 'anterior mitral leaflet'. This cleft is actually the separation between the left-sided portions of the primitive antero-superior and postero-inferior bridging leaflets. *see also* AVSD.

• ostium secundum ASD. Located at the level of the oval fossa.

• sinus venosus ASD. *see* sinus venosus defect.

atrial switch procedure

A procedure to redirect venous return to the contralateral ventricle. When used in complete transposition of the great arteries (either the Mustard or the Senning procedure) this accomplishes physiologic correction of the circulation, while leaving the right ventricle to support the systemic circulation. In patients with l-transposition of the great arteries and in patients who have had a previous Mustard or Senning procedure, it is used as part of a 'double switch procedure' which results in anatomic correction of the circulation, with the left ventricle supporting the systemic circulation. *see also* double switch procedure.

atrioventricular concordance

see concordant atrioventricular connections.

atrioventricular discordance

see discordant atrioventricular connections.

atrioventricular septal defect (AVSD)

A group of anomalies resulting from a deficiency of the atrioventricular septum which have in common: 1) a common atrioventricular junction with a common fibrous ring, and a unique, 5-leaflet, atrioventricular valve; 2) unwedging of the aorta from its usual position deeply wedged between the mitral and tricuspid valves; 3) a narrowed subaortic outflow tract; 4) disproportion between the inlet and outlet portions of the ventricular septum. Echocardiographic recognition is aided by the observation that 'left' and 'right' AV valves are located in the same anatomic plane. Included in this group of conditions are anomalies previously known as (and often still described as) ostium primum ASD (partial AVSD), 'cleft' anterior mitral and/or septal tricuspid valve leaflet, inlet VSD, and complete AVSD ('complete AV canal defect'). An older, obsolete, term describing such a defect is 'endocardial cushion defect'. *see also* endocardial cushion defect.

atrioventricular septum

The atrioventricular septum separates the left ventricular inlet from the right atrium. It has two parts: a muscular portion which exists because the attachment of the septal leaflet of the tricuspid valve is more towards the apex of the ventricle than the corresponding attachment of the mitral valve, and a fibrous portion superior to the attachment of the septal leaflet of the tricuspid valve. This latter portion separates the right atrium from the sub-aortic left ventricular outflow tract. *see also* Gerbode defect.

atrioventricular valve (AV valve)

A valve guarding the inlet to a ventricle. AV valves correspond with their respective ventricles, the tricuspid valve always associated with the right ventricle, and the mitral valve with the left ventricle. However, in the setting of an atrioventricular septal defect, there is neither a true mitral nor a true tricuspid valve. Rather, in severe forms there is a single atrioventricular orifice, guarded by a 5-leaflet AV valve. The 'left AV valve' comprises the left lateral leaflet and the left portions of the superior (anterior) and inferior (posterior) bridging leaflets, while the 'right AV valve' comprises the right inferior leaflet, the right antero-superior leaflet, and the right portions of the superior and inferior bridging leaflets.

• cleft AV valve. A defect often involving the left AV valve in AVSD formed by the conjunction of the superior and inferior bridging leaflets. A cleft may also be seen in the septal tricuspid leaflet. A similar but morphogenetically distinct entity may involve the anterior or rarely posterior leaflet of the mitral valve in otherwise normal hearts.

• common AV valve. Describes a 5-leaflet AV valve in complete AVSD that is related to both ventricles.

• overriding AV valve. Describes an AV valve that empties into both ventricles. It overrides the interventricular septum above a VSD.

- straddling AV valve. Describes an AV valve with anomalous insertion of tendinous cords or papillary muscles into the contralateral ventricle (VSD required).

autograft
Tissue or organ transplanted to a new site within the same individual.

AV septal defect (AVSD)
see atrioventricular septal defect (AVSD).

AV valve
see atrioventricular valve.

azygos continuation of the inferior vena cava
An anomaly of systemic venous connections wherein the inferior vena cava (IVC) is interrupted distal to its passage through the liver, and IVC flow reaches the right atrium through an enlarged azygos vein connecting the IVC to the superior vena cava. Usually, only hepatic venous flow reaches the right atrium from below. *see also* isomerism.

Baffes operation
Anastomosis of the right pulmonary veins to the right atrium (RA) and the IVC to the left atrium (LA) by using an allograft aortic tube to connect the IVC and the LA. (Baffes TG. A new method for surgical correction of transposition of the aorta and pulmonary artery. *Surg Gynecol Obstet* 1956, **102**, 227–233). This operation provided partial physiologic correction in patients with complete TGA. Lillehei and Varco originally described such a procedure in 1953. (Lillehei CW, Varco RL. Certain physiologic, pathologic, and surgical features of complete transposition of great vessels. *Surgery* 1953, **34**, 376–400.)

baffle
A structure surgically created to divert blood flow. For instance, in atrial switch operations for complete transposition of the great vessels, an intra-atrial baffle is constructed to divert systemic venous return across the mitral valve, thence to the left ventricle and pulmonary artery, and pulmonary venous return across the tricuspid valve, thence to the right ventricle and aorta. *see also* Mustard procedure. *see also* Senning procedure.

balanced
As in 'balanced circulation', e.g. in the setting of VSD and pulmonary stenosis. The pulmonary stenosis is such that there is neither excessive pulmonary blood flow (which might lead to pulmonary hypertension) nor inadequate pulmonary blood flow (which might lead to marked cyanosis). *see also* ventricular imbalance.

Bentall procedure

Replacement of the ascending aorta and the aortic valve with a composite graft-valve device and reimplantation of the coronary ostia into the sides of the conduit. (Bentall H, DeBono A. A technique for complete replacement of the ascending aorta. *Thorax* 1968, **23**, 338–339.)

• Exclusion technique: the native aorta is resected and replaced by the prosthetic graft.

• Inclusion technique: the walls of the native aorta are wrapped around the graft so that the prosthetic material is 'included'.

bicuspid aortic valve

An anomaly wherein the aortic valve is comprised of only two cusps instead of the usual three. There is often a raphe or aborted commissure dividing the larger cusp anatomically but not functionally. This anomaly is seen in 2% of the general population and in 75% of patents with aortic coarctation.

bidirectional cavopulmonary anastomosis

see Glenn shunt/bidirectional Glenn.

Björk modification

see Fontan procedure/RA-RV Fontan.

Blalock-Hanlon atrial septectomy

A palliative procedure to improve arterial oxygen saturation in patients with complete transposition of the great arteries, first described in 1950. A surgical atrial septectomy is accomplished through a right lateral thoracotomy, excising the posterior aspect of the interatrial septum to provide mixing of systemic and pulmonary venous return at the atrial level. (Blalock A, Hanlon CR. Surgical treatment of complete transposition of aorta and pulmonary artery. *Surg Gynecol Obstet* 1950, **90**, 1–15.)

Blalock-Taussig shunt

A palliative operation for the purpose of increasing pulmonary blood flow, hence systemic oxygen saturation. It involves creating an anastomosis between a subclavian artery and the ipsilateral pulmonary artery either directly with an end-to-side anastomosis (classical) or using an interposition tube graft (modified). (Blalock A, Taussig HB. The surgical treatment of malformations of the heart in which there is pulmonary stenosis or pulmonary atresia. *Journal of the American Medical Association* 1945, **128**, 189–202.)

Bland-White-Garland Syndrome

The left main coronary artery arises from the main pulmonary artery. The first report describing clinical and pathologic features was published in 1933. (Bland EF, White PD, Garland J. Congenital anomalies of the coronary arteries: report of an unusual case associated with cardiac hypertrophy. *American Heart Journal* 1933, **8**, 787; 801) *syn.* ALCAPA.

bridging leaflets

The superior and the inferior bridging leaflets of the AV valve are two leaflets uniquely found in association with AVSD. They 'bridge', or pass across, the interventricular septum. When the central part of the bridging leaflet tissue runs within the interventricular septum, the AV valve is functionally separated into left and right components. When the bridging leaflets do not run within the interventricular septum, but pass over its crest, a common AV valve guarding a common AV orifice (with an obligatory VSD) is the result.

Brock procedure

A palliative operation to increase pulmonary blood flow and reduce right-to-left shunting in tetralogy of Fallot. It involved resection of part of the right ventricle (RV) infundibulum using a punch or biopsy-like instrument introduced through the right ventricle so as to reduce RV outflow tract obstruction, without VSD closure. The operation was performed without cardiopulmonary bypass. (Brock RC. Pulmonary valvotomy for the relief of congenital pulmonary stenosis: report of three cases. *British Medical Journal* 1948, **1**, 1121–1126.)

bulbo-ventricular foramen

syn. primary foramen, primary ventricular foramen, primary interventricular foramen. An embryological term describing the connection between the left-sided inflow segments (primitive atrium and presumptive left ventricle) and the right-sided outflow segments (presumptive right ventricle and cono-truncus) in the primitive heart tube.

CACH (Canadian Adult Congenital Heart) Network

A co-operative nationwide association of Canadian cardiologists, cardiac surgeons and others, many of whom are situated in regional referral centers for adult congenital heart disease, dedicated to improving the care of ACHD patients. For more information, visit http://www.cachnet.org.

cardiac position

Position of the heart in the chest with regard to its location, and the orientation of its apex.
- cardiac location – location of the heart in the chest:
    - levoposition – to the left;
    - mesoposition – central;
    - dextroposition – to the right.
Cardiac location is affected by many factors including underlying cardiac malformation, abnormalities of mediastinal and thoracic structures, tumors, kyphoscoliosis, abnormalities of the diaphragm.
- cardiac orientation – the base to apex orientation of the heart:

- levocardia – apex directed to the left of the midline;
- mesocardia – apex oriented inferiorly in the midline;
- dextrocardia – apex directed to the right of the midline.

The base to apex axis of the heart is defined by the alignment of the ventricles and is independent of cardiac situs (sidedness). This axis is best described by echocardiography using the apical and subcostal 4-chamber views.

• cardiac sidedness. *see* situs.

cardiopulmonary study

A rest and stress study of cardiopulmonary physiology, including at least the following elements: resting pulmonary function, stress study to assess maximum workload, maximum oxygen uptake (MVO_2), anerobic threshold (AT), and oxygen saturation with effort.

Cardio-Seal® device

A device delivered percutaneously by catheter for closure of an ASD or PFO.

CATCH 22

Syndrome due to microdeletion at chromosome 22q11 resulting in a wide clinical spectrum. CATCH stands for **C**ardiac defect, **A**bnormal facies, **T**hymic hypoplasia, **C**left palate, and **H**ypocalcemia. Cardiac defects include cono-truncal defects such as interrupted aortic arch, tetralogy of Fallot, truncus arteriosus, and double outlet right ventricle. *see also* DiGeorge syndrome, velo-cardio-facial syndrome.

cat's eye syndrome

A syndrome due to a tandem duplication of chromosome 22q or an isodicentric chromosome 22 such that the critical region 22pter – > q11 is duplicated. Phenotypic features include mental deficiency, anal and renal malformations, hypertelorism and others. Total anomalous pulmonary venous return is the commonest congenital cardiac lesion (in up to 40% of patients).

CHARGE association

This anomaly is characterized by the presence of coloboma or choanal atresia and three of the following defects: congenital heart disease, nervous system anomaly or mental retardation, genital abnormalities, ear abnormality or deafness. If coloboma and choanal atresia are both present, only two of the additional (minor) abnormalities are needed for diagnosis. Congenital heart defects seen in the CHARGE association are: tetralogy of Fallot with or without other cardiac defects, atrioventricular septal defect, double outlet right ventricle, double inlet left ventricle, transposition of the great arteries, interrupted aortic arch and others.

Chiari network

Fenestrated remnant of the right valve of the sinus venosus resulting from incomplete regression of this structure during embryogenesis and first described in 1897 (Chiari H. Ueber Netzbildungen im rechten Vorhof. *Beitr Pathol Anat* 1897, **22**, 1–10). The prevalence is 2% in autopsy and echocardiography studies. It presents with coarse right atrial reticula connected to the Eustachian and Thebesian valves and attached to the crista terminalis. It may be associated with patent foramen ovale and interatrial septal aneurysm.

cleft AV valve

see atrioventricular valve; *see also* atrial septal defect. *see also* ostium primum ASD.

coarctation of the aorta

A stenosis of the proximal descending aorta varying in anatomy, physiology and clinical presentation. It may present with discrete or long-segment stenosis, is frequently associated with hypoplasia of the aortic arch and bicuspid aortic valve and may be part of a Shone complex.

common (as in: AV valve, atrium, ventricle, etc.)

Implies bilateral structures with absent septation. Contrasts with 'single', which implies absence of corresponding contralateral structure. *see also* single.

common atrium

Large atrium characterized by a nonrestrictive communication between the bilateral atria due to the absence of most of the atrial septum. Frequently associated with complex congenital heart disease (isomerism, atrioventricular septal defect, etc.). *see also* single (atrium).

common arterial trunk

see truncus arteriosus.

complete transposition of the great arteries

syn. classic transposition; d-transposition; d-TGA; atrioventricular concordance with ventriculo-arterial discordance. An anomaly wherein the aorta arises from the right ventricle and the pulmonary artery arises from the left ventricle. The right ventricle supports the systemic circulation.

concordant atrioventricular connections

Appropriate connection of morphologic right atrium to morphologic right ventricle and of morphologic left atrium to morphologic left ventricle. *syn.* atrioventricular concordance.

concordant ventriculo-arterial connections
Appropriate origin of pulmonary trunk from morphologic right ventricle and of aorta from morphologic left ventricle. *syn.* ventriculo-arterial concordance.

conduit
A structure that connects non-adjacent parts of the cardiovascular system, allowing blood to flow between them. Often fashioned from prosthetic material. May include a valve.

congenital coronary arteriovenous fistula (CCAVF)
A direct communication between a coronary artery and cardiac chamber, great artery or vena cava, bypassing the coronary capillary network.

congenital heart disease (CHD)
Anomalies of the heart originating in fetal life. Their expression may, however, be delayed beyond the neonatal period, and may change with time as further postnatal physiologic and anatomic changes occur.

congenitally corrected transposition of the great arteries
syn. cc-TGA; l-transposition; l-TGA; atrioventricular discordance with ventriculo-arterial discordance; double discordance. An anomaly wherein the aorta arises from the right ventricle and the pulmonary artery from the left ventricle, and, in addition, the atrioventricular connection is discordant such that the right atrium connects to the left ventricle and the left atrium connects to the right ventricle. There are usually associated anomalies, the most common being ventricular septal defect, pulmonic stenosis, and/or a hypoplastic ventricle. The right ventricle supports the systemic circulation.

congenital pericardial defect
A defect in the pericardium due to defective formation of the pleuro-pericardial membrane of the septum transversum. The spectrum of pericardial deficiency is wide. It may be partial or total. Its clinical diagnosis is difficult. Left-sided defects are more common. Total absence of the pericardium may be associated with other defects such as bronchogenic cyst, pulmonary sequestration, hypoplastic lung, and other congenital heart diseases.

connection
Anatomic link between two structures (e.g. veno-atrial, atrioventricular, ventriculo-arterial).

cono-truncal abnormality
Neural crest cell migration is crucial for cono-truncal septation and the development of both the pulmonary and aortic outflow tracts. If neural crest cell migration fails, cono-truncal abnormalities occur. The most common cono-truncal anomalies are truncus arteriosus and interrupted aortic arch. Other defects may

include tetralogy of Fallot, pulmonary atresia with ventricular septal defect, absent pulmonary valve or d-malposition of the great arteries with double outlet right ventricle, single ventricle or tricuspid atresia. Abnormal neural crest migration may also be associated with complex clinical entities, such as CATCH 22.

conus
see infundibulum.

cor triatriatum sinister
A membrane divides the left atrium into an accessory pulmonary venous chamber and a left atrial chamber contiguous with the mitral valve. The pulmonary veins enter the accessory chamber. The connection between the accessory chamber and the true left atrium varies in size and may produce pulmonary venous obstruction.

cor triatriatum dexter
Abnormal septation of the right atrium due to failure of regression of the right valve of the sinus venosus. This yields a smooth-walled posteromedial 'sinus' chamber (embryologic origin of the sinus venosus) that receives the venae cavae and (usually) the coronary sinus, and a trabeculated anterolateral 'atrial' chamber (embryologic origin of the primitive right atrium) that includes the right atrial appendage and is related to the tricuspid valve. Usually, there is free communication between these two compartments, but variable obstruction to systemic venous flow from the 'sinus' chamber to the 'atrial' chamber may occur and may be associated with underdevelopment of downstream right heart structures (e.g. hypoplastic tricuspid valve, tricuspid atresia, pulmonary stenosis or pulmonary atresia). A patent foramen ovale or an atrial septal defect are often present in relation to the posteromedial chamber.

When there is more extensive resorption of the right valve of the sinus venosus, remnants form the Eustachian valve related to the inferior vena cava, the Thebesian valve related to the coronary sinus, and the crista terminalis. Chiari network describes right atrial reticula, which are extensively fenestrated remnants of the right sinus venosus valve. *see* sinus venosus.

criss-cross heart
syn. criss-cross atrioventricular connection. A rotational abnormality of the ventricular mass around its long axis resulting in relationships of the ventricular chambers not anticipated from the given atrioventricular connections. If the rotated ventricles are in a markedly supero-inferior relationship, the heart may also be described as a supero-inferior or upstairs-downstairs heart. There may be ventriculo-arterial concordance or discordance.

crista supraventricularis
A saddle-shaped muscular crest in the right ventricular outflow tract intervening between the tricuspid valve and the pulmonary valve, consisting of septal

and parietal components, which demarcates the junction between the outlet septum and the pulmonary infundibulum. Occasionally, but less accurately termed crista ventricularis.

crista terminalis
A vestigial remnant of the right valve of the sinus venosus located at the junction of the trabeculated right atrial appendage and the smooth-walled 'sinus' component of the right atrium component receiving the inferior vena cava, the superior vena cava, and the coronary sinus. A feature of right atrial internal anatomy. *syn.* terminal crest.

crista ventricularis
see crista supraventricularis.

cyanosis
A bluish discoloration due to the presence of an increased quantity of desaturated hemoglobin in tissues. In congenital heart disease, cyanosis is generally due to right-to-left shunting through congenital cardiac defects, bypassing the pulmonary alveoli, or due to acquired intrapulmonary shunts (central cyanosis). Cyanosis can also occur due to increased peripheral extraction due, for instance, to critically reduced cutaneous flow (peripheral cyanosis).

Dacron®
A synthetic material often used to fashion conduits and other prosthetic devices for the surgical palliation or repair of congenital heart disease.

Damus-Kaye-Stansel operation
A procedure reserved for patients with abnormal ventriculo-arterial connections who are not suitable for an arterial switch operation (e.g. TGA and non-suitable coronary patterns, DORV with severe subaortic stenosis, systemic ventricular outflow tract obstruction in hearts with a univentricular AV connection). The operation involves anastomosis of the proximal end of the transected main pulmonary artery in an end-to-side fashion to the ascending aorta to provide blood flow from the systemic ventricle to the aorta; coronary arteries are not translocated and are perfused in a retrograde fashion. The aortic orifice and a VSD (if present) are closed with a patch. A conduit between the right ventricle and the distal pulmonary artery provides venous blood to the lungs. The procedure was described in 1975. (Damus PS. Correspondence. *Annals of Thoracic Surgery* 1975, **20**, 724–725.) (Kaye MP. Anatomic correction of transposition of the great arteries. *Mayo Clinic Proceedings* 1975, **50**, 638–640.) (Stansel HC Jr. A new operation for d-loop transposition of the great vessels. *Annals of Thoracic Surgery* 1975, **19**, 565–567.)

David operation

A surgical procedure for ascending aortic aneurysm, involving replacement of the ascending aorta with a synthetic tube and remodeling of the aortic root so the preserved aortic valve is no longer regurgitant (David TE, Feindel CM. An aortic valve sparing operation for patients with aortic incompetence and aneurysm of the ascending aorta. *Journal of Thoracic and Cardiovascular Surgery* 1992, **103**, 617–621.)

dextrocardia

Cardiac apex directed to the right of the midline. *see* cardiac position.

dextroposition

Rightward shift of the heart. *see* cardiac position.

dextroversion

An old term for dextrocardia. *see* cardiac position.

differential hypoxemia; differential cyanosis

A difference in the degree of hypoxemia/cyanosis in different extremities as a result of the site of a right-to-left shunt. The most common situation is of greater hypoxemia/cyanosis in feet and sometimes left hand, as compared to right hand and head, in a patient with an Eisenmenger PDA.

DiGeorge syndrome

An autosomal dominant syndrome now known to be part of 'CATCH 22'. As originally described, it consisted of infantile hypocalcemia, immunodeficiency due to thymic hypoplasia, and a cono-truncal cardiac abnormality. *see also* CATCH 22.

discordant atrioventricular connections

Anomalous connection of atria and ventricles such that the morphologic right atrium connects via a mitral valve to a morphologic left ventricle, while the morphologic left atrium connects via a tricuspid valve to a morphologic right ventricle.

discordant ventriculo-arterial connections

Anomalous connection of the great arteries and ventricles such that the pulmonary trunk arises from the left ventricle and the aorta arises from the right ventricle.

diverticulum of Kommerell

Enlarged origin of the left subclavian artery associated with right aortic arch. Its diameter may be equal to that of the descending aorta and tapers to the left subclavian diameter. It is found at the origin of the aberrant left subclavian artery, the fourth branch off the right aortic arch.

double aortic arch
see aortic arch anomaly.

double-chambered RV
Separation of the right ventricle (RV) into a higher-pressure inflow chamber, and a lower pressure infundibular chamber, the separation usually being produced by hypertrophy of the 'septomarginal band'. When a VSD is present, it usually communicates with the high pressure RV inflow chamber.

double discordance
see congenitally corrected transposition of the great arteries.

double inlet left ventricle (DILV)
see univentricular connection.

double orifice mitral valve
The mitral valve orifice is partially or completely divided into two parts by a fibrous bridge of tissue. Both orifices enter the left ventricle. Mitral regurgitation and/or mitral stenosis may be present. Aortic coarctation and atrioventricular septal defect are commonly associated defects.

double outlet left ventricle (DOLV)
Both the pulmonary artery and the aorta arise predominantly from the morphologic left ventricle. DOLV is rare, and much less frequent than double outlet right ventricle (DORV).

double outlet right ventricle (DORV)
Both great arteries arise predominantly from the morphologic right ventricle; there is usually no fibrous continuity between the semilunar and the AV valves; a ventricular septal defect is present. When the VSD is in the subaortic position without RV outflow tract obstruction, the physiology simulates a simple VSD. With RV outflow tract obstruction, the physiology simulates tetralogy of Fallot. When the VSD is in the subpulmonary position (the Taussig-Bing anomaly), the physiology simulates complete transposition of the great arteries with VSD. *see also* Taussig-Bing anomaly.

double switch procedure
An operation used in patients with l-transposition of the great arteries (l-TGA; congenitally corrected transposition of the great arteries; cc-TGA) and also in patients who have had a prior Mustard or Senning atrial switch operation for complete transposition of the great arteries (d-TGA). It leads to anatomic correction of the ventricle to great artery relationships such that the left ventricle

supports the systemic circulation. It includes an arterial switch procedure (*see* Jatene operation) in all cases, as well as an atrial switch procedure (Mustard or Senning) in the case of l-TGA, or reversal of the previously done Mustard or Senning procedure in the case of d-TGA.

doubly-committed VSD
see ventricular septal defect.

Down syndrome
The most common malformation caused by trisomy 21. Most of the patients (95%) have complete trisomy of chromosome 21; some have translocation or mosaic forms. The phenotype is diagnostic (short stature, characteristic facial appearance, mental retardation, brachydactyly, atlanto-axial instability, thyroid and white blood cell disorders). Congenital heart defects are frequent, atrioventricular septal defect and ventricular septal defect being the most common. Mitral valve prolapse and aortic regurgitation may be present. Down syndrome patients are prone to earlier and more severe pulmonary vascular disease than might otherwise be expected as a consequence of the lesions identified.

dural ectasia
Expansion of the dural sac in the lumbo-sacral area, seen on CT or MRI. It is one of the criteria used to confirm the diagnosis of Marfan syndrome. (Pyeritz RE, *et al.* Dural ectasia is a common feature of the Marfan syndrome *American Journal of Human Genetics* 1988, **43**, 726–732.) (Fattori R, *et al.* Importance of dural ectasia in phenotypic assessment of Marfan's syndrome. *Lancet* 1999, **354**, 910–913.)

Ebstein anomaly
An anomaly of the tricuspid valve in which the basal attachments of both the septal and the posterior valve leaflets are displaced apically within the right ventricle. Apical displacement of the septal tricuspid leaflet of >8 mm/M2 is diagnostic (the extent of apical displacement should be indexed to body surface area). Abnormal structure of all three leaflets is seen, with the anterior leaflet typically large with abnormal attachments to the right ventricular wall. The pathologic and clinical spectrum is broad and includes not only valve abnormalities but also myocardial structural changes in both ventricles. Tricuspid regurgitation is common, tricuspid stenosis occurs occasionally, and right-to-left shunting through a patent foramen ovale or atrial septal defect is a regular but not invariable concomitant. Other congenital lesions are often associated, such as VSD, pulmonary stenosis, and/or accessory conduction pathways.

Ehlers-Danlos syndrome (EDS)
A group of heritable disorders of connective tissue, (specifically, abnormalities of collagen). Hyperextensibility of the joints and hyperelasticity and fragility of the skin are common to all forms; patients bruise easily.

• Ehlers-Danlos types I, II and III, which demonstrate autosomal dominant inheritance, are the commonest forms, each representing about 30% of cases. The cardiovascular abnormalities are generally mild, consisting of mitral and tricuspid valve prolapse. Dilatation of major arteries, including the aorta, may occur. Aortic rupture is seen rarely in type I, but not in types II and III.

• Ehlers-Danlos syndrome type IV is also autosomal dominant, but frequently appears de novo. This is the 'arterial' form, presenting with aortic dilatation and rupture of medium and large arteries spontaneously or after trauma. It is due to an abnormality of type III procollagen, and comprises about 10% of cases of Ehlers-Danlos syndrome.

• There are 6 other rare types of Ehlers-Danlos syndrome.

Eisenmenger syndrome
An extreme form of pulmonary vascular obstructive disease arising as a consequence of pre-existing systemic to pulmonary shunt, wherein pulmonary vascular resistance rises such that pulmonary pressures are at or near systemic levels and there is reversed (right-to-left) or bidirectional shunting at great vessel, ventricular, and/or atrial levels. *see also* Heath-Edwards classification. *see also* pulmonary hypertension.

Ellis-van Creveld syndrome
An autosomal recessive syndrome in which common atrium, primum ASD and partial AV septal defect are the most common cardiac lesions.

endocardial cushion defect
see atrioventricular septal defect. The term endocardial cushion defect has fallen into disuse because it implies an outdated concept of the morphogenesis of the atrioventricular septum.

erythrocytosis
Increase in red blood cell concentration secondary to chronic tissue hypoxia, as seen in cyanotic CHD and in chronic pulmonary disease. It results from a hypoxia-induced physiologic response resulting in increased erythropoietin levels, and affects only the red cell line. It is also called secondary erythrocytosis. The term 'polycythemia' is inaccurate in this context, since other blood cell lines are not affected. *see also* polycythemia vera. Erythrocytosis may cause hyperviscosity symptoms. *see also* hyperviscosity.

Eustachian valve
A remnant of the right valve of the sinus venosus guarding the entrance of the inferior vena cava to the right atrium.

extracardiac Fontan
see Fontan procedure.

fenestration
An opening, or 'window' (usually small) between two structures, which may be spontaneous, traumatic, or created surgically.

fibrillin
Fibrillin is a large glycoprotein, closely involved with collagen in the structure of connective tissue. Mutations in the fibrillin gene on chromosome 15 are responsible for all manifestations of Marfan syndrome. *see also* Marfan syndrome.

Fontan procedure (operation)
A palliative operation for patients with a univentricular circulation, involving diversion of the systemic venous return to the pulmonary artery, usually without the interposition of a subpulmonary ventricle. There are many variations, all leading to normalization of systemic oxygen saturation and elimination of volume overload of the functioning ventricle.
• classic Fontan. Originally, a valved conduit between the right atrium and the pulmonary artery (Fontan F, Baudet E. Surgical repair of tricuspid atresia. *Thorax* 1971, **26**, 240–248.) Subsequently changed to a direct anastomosis between right atrium (RA) and pulmonary artery (PA).
• extracardiac Fontan. Inferior vena cava (IVC) blood is directed to the pulmonary artery via an extracardiac conduit. The superior vena cava (SVC) is anastomosed to the PA as in the bidirectional Glenn shunt.
• fenestrated Fontan. Surgical creation of an ASD in the atrial patch or baffle to provide an escape valve, allowing right-to-left shunting to reduce pressure in the systemic venous circuit, at the expense of systemic hypoxemia.
• lateral tunnel. *see* total cavopulmonary connection (TCPC).
• RA-RV Fontan. Conduit (often valved) between right atrium (RA) and right ventricle (RV). Also known as the Björk modification. (Björk VO, *et al.* Right atrial-ventricular anastomosis for correction of tricuspid atresia. *Journal of Thoracic and Cardiovascular Surgery* 1979, **77**, 452–458.)
• total cavopulmonary connection (TCPC). IVC flow is directed by a baffle within the RA into the lower portion of the divided SVC or the right atrial appendage, which is connected to the pulmonary artery. The upper part of the SVC is connected to the superior aspect of the pulmonary artery as in the bidirectional Glenn procedure. The majority of the RA is excluded from the systemic venous circuit. *syn.* lateral tunnel Fontan.

Gerbode defect
An unusual variant of atrioventricular septal defect, wherein the defect is in the superior portion of the atrioventricular septum above the insertion of the septal leaflet of the tricuspid valve, resulting in a direct communication and shunt between the left ventricle and the right atrium. *see also* atrioventricular septum.

Ghent criteria

A set of criteria for the diagnosis of Marfan syndrome, requiring involvement of three organ systems (one system must have 'major' involvement), or two organ systems and a positive family history. (DePaepe A, Deitz HC, Devereux RB, *et al.* Revised diagnostic criteria for the Marfan syndrome. *American Journal of Medical Genetics* 1996, **62**, 417–426)

Glenn shunt (operation)

A palliative operation for the purpose of increasing pulmonary blood flow, hence systemic oxygen saturation, in which a direct anastomosis is created between the superior vena cava (SVC) and a pulmonary artery (PA). This procedure does not cause systemic ventricular volume overload.

• classic Glenn. Anastomosis of the SVC to the distal end of the divided right PA with division/ligation of the SVC below the anastomosis. Acquired pulmonary arterio-venous malformations with associated systemic arterial desaturation are a common long-term complication. (Glenn WW. Circulatory bypass of the right side of the heart. IV. Shunt between superior vena cava and distal right pulmonary artery: report of clinical application. *New England Journal of Medicine* 1958, **259**, 117–120.)

• bidirectional Glenn. End-to-side anastomosis of the divided SVC to the undivided PA. (Haller JA Jr, *et al.* Experimental studies in permanent bypass of the right heart. *Surgery* 1966, **59**, 1128–1132.) (Azzolina G, *et al.* Tricuspid atresia: experience in surgical management with a modified cavopulmonary anastomosis. *Thorax* 1972, **27**, 111–115.) (Hopkins RA *et al.* Physiologic rationale for a bi-directional cavopulmonary shunt. A versatile complement to the Fontan principle. *Journal of Thoracic and Cardiovascular Surgery* 1985, **90**, 391–398.)

Gore-Tex®

A synthetic material often used to fashion conduits and other prosthetic devices for the surgical palliation or repair of congenital heart disease.

GUCH

Grown-up congenital heart disease. A term originated by Dr Jane Somerville. *syn.* Adult congenital heart disease

Heath-Edwards classification

A histopathologic classification useful in assessing the potential for reversibility of pulmonary vascular disease. (Heath D, Edwards JE. The pathology of hypertensive pulmonary vascular disease: A description of six grades of structural changes in the pulmonary arteries with special reference to congenital cardiac septal defects. *Circulation* 1958, **18**, 533–547.)

• Grade I – hypertrophy of the media of small muscular arteries and arterioles.

• Grade II – intimal cellular proliferation in addition to medial hypertrophy.

- Grade III – advanced medial thickening with hypertrophy and hyperplasia including progressive intimal proliferation and concentric fibrosis. This results in obliteration of arterioles and small arteries.
- Grade IV – 'plexiform lesions' of the muscular pulmonary arteries and arterioles with a plexiform network of capillary-like channels within a dilated segment.
- Grade V – complex plexiform, angiomatous and cavernous lesions and hyalinization of intimal fibrosis.
- Grade VI – necrotizing arteritis.

hemi-Fontan
The first part of a 'staged Fontan', sometimes chosen to reduce the morbidity and mortality that might be associated with performing the complete Fontan at one operation. The hemi-Fontan includes a bidirectional cavopulmonary anastomosis and obliteration of central shunts. The second step to complete the Fontan procedure may be performed at a later time.

hemi-truncus
An anomalous pulmonary artery branch to one lung arising from the ascending aorta in the presence of a main pulmonary artery arising normally from the right ventricle and supplying the other lung.

heterograft
Transplanted tissue or organ from a different species.

heterotaxy
Abnormal arrangement (*taxo* in Greek) of viscera that differs from the arrangement seen in either situs solitus or situs inversus. Often described as 'visceral heterotaxy'.

heterotopic
Located in an anatomically abnormal site, often in reference to transplantation of an organ.

Holt-Oram syndrome
Autosomal dominant syndrome consisting of radial abnormalities of the forearm and hand associated with secundum ASD (most common), VSD, or, rarely, other cardiac malformations. (Holt M, Oram S. Familial heart disease with skeletal manifestations. *British Heart Journal* 1960, **22**, 236–242.) The gene for this syndrome is on 12q2. (Basson CT, *et al*. The clinical and genetic spectrum of the Holt-Oram syndrome [heart-hand syndrome] *New England Journal of Medicine* 1994, **330**, 885–891.)

homograft
Transplanted tissue or organ from another individual of the same species.

Hunter syndrome

A genetic syndrome due to a deficiency of the enzyme iduronate sulfate (mucopolysaccharidase) with X-linked recessive inheritance. Clinical spectrum is wide. Patients present with skeletal changes, mental retardation, arterial hypertension and involvement of atrioventricular and semilunar valves resulting in valve regurgitation.

Hurler syndrome

A genetic syndrome due to a deficiency of the enzyme a-L-iduronidase (mucopolysaccharidase) with autosomal recessive inheritance. Phenotype presents with a wide spectrum including severe skeletal abnormalities, corneal clouding, hepatosplenomegaly, mental retardation and mitral valve stenosis.

hyperviscosity

An excessive increase in viscosity of blood, as may occur secondary to erythrocytosis in patients with cyanotic congenital heart disease. Hyperviscosity symptoms include: headache; impaired alertness, depressed mentation or a sense of distance; visual disturbances (blurred vision, double vision, amaurosis fugax); paresthesiae of fingers, toes or lips; tinnitus; fatigue, lassitude; myalgias (including chest, abdominal muscles), and muscle weakness. (Perloff JK, *et al.* Adults with cyanotic congenital heart disease: hematologic management. *Annals of Internal Medicine* 1988, **109**, 406–413.) Restless legs or a sensation of cold legs may reflect hyperviscosity (observation of Dr E. Oechslin). As the symptoms are non-specific, their relation to hyperviscosity is supported if they are alleviated by phlebotomy. Iron deficiency and dehydration worsen hyperviscosity and must be avoided, or treated if present.

hypoplastic left heart syndrome

A heterogeneous syndrome with a wide variety and severity of manifestations involving hypoplasia, stenosis, or atresia at different levels of the left heart including the aorta, aortic valve, left ventricular outflow tract, left ventricular body, mitral valve and left atrium.

Ilbawi procedure (operation)

An operation for congenitally corrected transposition of the great arteries with VSD and pulmonary stenosis, wherein a communication is established between the left ventricle (LV) and the aorta via the VSD using a baffle within the right ventricle (RV). The RV is connected to the pulmonary artery using a valved conduit. An atrial switch procedure is done. The LV then supports the systemic circulation. (Ilbawi MN, *et al.* An alternative approach to the surgical management of physiologically corrected transposition with ventricular septal defect and pulmonary stenosis or atresia. *Journal of Thoracic and Cardiovascular Surgery* 1990, **100**, 410–415.)

infracristal
Located below the crista supraventricularis in the right ventricular outflow tract. *see* crista supraventricularis.

infundibular, infundibulum
(Pertaining to) a ventricular-great arterial connecting segment. Normally sub-pulmonary, but can be sub-aortic, and may be bilateral or absent. Bilateral infundibulum may be seen in patients with TGA/VSD/pulmonary stenosis (PS), DORV with VSD/PS, and anatomically corrected malposition. *syn.* conus.

inlet VSD
see ventricular septal defect.

interrupted aortic arch
see aortic arch anomaly.

interrupted inferior vena cava
The inferior vena cava is interrupted below the hepatic veins with subsequent systemic venous drainage via the azygos vein to the superior vena cava. The hepatic veins enter the right atrium directly. This anomaly is frequently associated with complex congenital heart disease, particularly left-isomerism.

ISACCD
International Society for Adult Congenital Cardiac Disease. For information link through http://www.isaccd.org

isolation of arch vessels
see aortic arch anomalies.

isomerism
Paired, mirror image sets of normally single or non-identical organ systems (atria, lungs, and viscera), often associated with other abnormalities.
- right isomerism. *syn.* asplenia syndrome. Congenital syndrome consisting of paired morphologically right structures: absence of spleen, bilateral right bronchi, bilateral tri-lobed (right) lungs, two morphologic right atria, and multiple anomalies of systemic and pulmonary venous connections and other complex cardiac and non-cardiac anomalies.
- left isomerism. *syn.* polysplenia syndrome. A congenital syndrome consisting of paired, morphologically left structures: multiple bilateral spleens, bilateral left bronchi, bilateral bilobed (left) lungs, midline liver, two morphologic left atria, and complex congenital heart disease and other associated non-cardiac malformations.

Jatene procedure (operation)

syn. arterial switch procedure. An operation used in complete transposition of the great arteries, involving removal of the aorta from its attachment to the right ventricle, and of the pulmonary artery from the left ventricle, and the reattachment of the great arteries to the contralateral ventricles, with reimplantation of the coronary arteries into the neo-aorta. As a consequence, the left ventricle supports the systemic circulation. (Jatene AD, *et al.* Anatomic correction of transposition of the great vessels. *Journal of Thoracic and Cardiovascular Surgery* 1976, **72**, 364–370.) *see also* Lecompte manoeuvre.

juxtaposition of atrial appendages

A rare anomaly seen in patients with transposition of the great arteries and other complex congenital heart defects (dextrocardia, tricuspid atresia, etc.), wherein the atrial appendages are situated side by side. The right atrial appendage passes immediately behind the transposed main pulmonary artery in patients with leftward juxtaposition of atrial appendages.

Kartagener syndrome

Autosomal recessive syndrome consisting of situs inversus totalis, dextrocardia and defect of ciliary motility leading to sinusitis, bronchiectasis and sperm immobility. (Kartegener M. Zur Pathogenese der Bronchiektasien: Bronchiektasien bei Situs viscerum inversus. *Beitr Klinik Tuberkul* 1933, **28**, 231–234.) (Kartagener M, *et al.* Bronchiectasis with situs inversus. *Archives of Pediatrics* 1962, **79**, 193–196.) (Miller RD, *et al.* Kartagener's syndrome. *Chest* 1972, **62**, 130–136.)

Kommerell

see diverticulum of Kommerell.

Konno procedure (operation)

Repair of tunnel-like subvalvar LVOTO by aorto-ventriculoplasty. The operation involves enlargement of the left ventricular outflow tract by inserting a patch in the ventricular septum, as well as aortic valve replacement and enlargement of the aortic annulus and ascending aorta. (Konno S, *et al.* A new method for prosthetic valve replacement in congenital aortic stenosis associated with hypoplasia of the aortic valve ring. *Journal of Thoracic and Cardiovascular Surgery* 1975, **70**, 909–917.). In severe forms of LVOTO, a prosthetic-valve-containing conduit may be inserted between the left ventricular apex and descending aorta. (Didonato RM, *et al.* Left ventricular-aortic conduits in paediatric patients. *Journal of Thoracic and Cardiovascular Surgery* 1984, **88**, 82–91.) (Frommelt PC, *et al.* Natural history of apical left ventricular to aortic conduits in paediatric patients. *Circulation* 1991, **84** (Suppl III), 213–218.)

Lecompte manoeuvre
The pulmonary artery is brought anterior to the aorta during an arterial switch procedure in patients with d-transposition of the great arteries. *see also* Jatene procedure.

LEOPARD syndrome
This autosomal dominant condition includes **L**entigines, **E**KG abnormalities, **O**cular hypertelorism, **P**ulmonary stenosis, **A**bnormal genitalia, **R**etardation of growth, and **D**eafness. Rarely, cardiomyopathy or complex congenital heart disease may be present.

levocardia
Leftward-oriented cardiac apex (normal). *see* cardiac position.

levoposition
Leftward shift of the heart. *see* cardiac position.

ligamentum arteriosum
A normal fibrous structure that is the residuum of the ductus arteriosus after its spontaneous closure.

long-QT syndrome
Abnormal prolongation of QT-duration with subsequent risk for torsade de pointes, syncope and sudden cardiac death. It may be congenital or acquired (medications such as antiarrhythmics, antihistamines, some antibiotics; electrolyte disturbances such as hypocalcemia, hypomagnesemia, hypokalemia; hypothyroidism; and other factors.). QT-interval must be adjusted to heart rate.

looping
Bending of the primitive heart tube (normally to the right, dextro, d-) that determines the atrioventricular relationship.
• d-loop. Morphologic right ventricle lies to the right of the morphologic left ventricle (normal rightward bend).
• l-loop. Morphologic right ventricle lies to the left of the morphologic left ventricle (leftward bend).

Lutembacher syndrome
Atrial septal defect associated with mitral valve stenosis. The mitral valve stenosis is usually acquired (rheumatic).

LVOTO
Left ventricular outflow tract obstruction.

maladie de Roger
Eponymous designation for a small restrictive ventricular septal defect that is not associated with significant left ventricular volume overload or elevated pulmonary artery pressure. There is a loud VSD murmur due to the high velocity turbulent left-to-right shunt across the defect.

malposition
An abnormality of cardiac position. *see* cardiac position.

MAPCA
Major aorto-pulmonary collateral artery. A large abnormal arterial vessel arising from the aorta, connecting to a pulmonary artery (usually in the pulmonary hilum) and providing blood supply to the lungs. Found in complex pulmonary atresia and other complex CHD associated with severe reduction or absence of antegrade pulmonary blood flow from the ventricle(s).

Marfan syndrome
A connective tissue disorder with autosomal dominant inheritance caused by a defect in the fibrillin gene on chromosome 15. The phenotypic expression varies. Patients may have tall stature, abnormal body proportions, ocular abnormalities, dural ectasia, protrusio acetabulae, and present with skeletal and cardiovascular abnormalities. Mitral valve prolapse with mitral regurgitation, ascending aortic dilatation/aneurysm with subsequent aortic regurgitation, and aortic dissection are the most common cardiovascular abnormalities. *see also* Ghent criteria.

mesocardia
Cardiac apex directed to mid-chest. *see* cardiac position.

mesoposition
Shift of the heart toward the midline. *see* cardiac position.

mitral arcade
Chordae of the mitral valve are shortened or absent and the thickened mitral valve leaflets insert directly into the papillary muscle ('hammock valve'). Mitral valve excursion is limited and results in mitral stenosis.

moderator band
A prominent muscular structure traversing the right ventricle from the base of the anterior papillary muscle to the septum near the apex.

muscular VSD
see ventricular septal defect.

Mustard procedure (operation)

An operation for complete transposition of the great arteries, in which venous return is directed to the contralateral ventricle by means of an atrial baffle made from autologous pericardial tissue or (rarely) synthetic material, after resection of most of the atrial septum. As a consequence, the right ventricle supports the systemic circulation. A type of 'atrial switch' operation (*see also* Senning procedure, atrial switch procedure, double switch procedure). (Mustard WT. Successful two-stage correction of transposition of the great vessels. *Surgery* 1964, **55**, 469–472.)

national referral center

see supraregional referral center (SRRC).

nonrestrictive VSD

see ventricular septal defect.

Noonan syndrome

An autosomal dominant syndrome phenotypically somewhat similar to Turner syndrome, with a normal chromosomal complement, due to an abnormality in chromosome 12q. It is associated with congenital cardiac anomalies, especially dysplastic pulmonic valve stenosis, pulmonary artery stenosis, ASD, tetralogy of Fallot, or hypertrophic cardiomyopathy. Congenital lymphedema is a common associated anomaly that may be unrecognized. (Noonan JA, Ehmke DA. Associated non-cardiac malformations in children with congenital heart disease. *Midwest Society for Pediatric Research* 1963, **63**, 468.)

Norwood procedure

A multistage operation for hypoplastic left heart syndrome. A systemic to pulmonary arterial shunt is created, followed by a staged Fontan-type operation (usually via a hemi-Fontan procedure) resulting in single ventricle physiology. The morphologic right ventricle supports the systemic circulation.

orthotopic

Located in an anatomically normal recipient site, often in reference to transplantation of an organ.

ostium primum ASD

see atrial septal defect.

outlet VSD

see ventricular septal defect.

over-and-under ventricles

see supero-inferior heart.

overriding valve
An AV valve that empties into both ventricles or a semilunar valve that origi-
nates from both ventricles.

palliation, palliative operation
A procedure carried out for the purpose of relieving symptoms or ameliorat-
ing some of the adverse effects of an anomaly, which does not address the
fundamental anatomic/physiologic disturbance. Contrasts with 'repair' or 'reparative operation'.

PAPVC
Partial anomalous pulmonary venous connection. *see* anomalous pulmonary
venous connection.

parachute mitral valve
A mitral valve abnormality in which all chordae tendineae of the mitral valve,
which may be shortened and thickened, insert in a single, abnormal papillary
muscle, usually causing mitral stenosis. The parachute mitral valve may be
part of the Shone complex. *see also* Shone complex.

partial AV septal defect
see atrioventricular septal defect

patent ductus arteriosus (PDA)
A ductus that fails to undergo normal closure in the early postnatal period.
syn: persistently patent ductus arteriosus, persistent arterial duct.

patent foramen ovale (PFO)
Failure of anatomic fusion of the valve of the foramen ovale with the limbus
of the fossa ovalis that normally occurs when left atrial pressure exceeds right
atrial pressure after birth. There is no structural deficiency of tissue of the
atrial septum. The foramen is functionally closed as long as left atrial pressure
exceeds right atrial pressure, but can reopen if right atrial pressure rises. Patent foramen ovale is found in up to 35% of the adult population in pathological
studies. The lower and variable prevalence reported in clinical series depends
on the techniques used to find it. *syn:* probe-patent foramen ovale, PFO.

pentalogy of Fallot
Tetralogy of Fallot with, in addition, an ASD or PFO. *see* tetralogy of Fallot.

perimembranous VSD
see ventricular septal defect.

persistent left superior vena cava (LSVC)
Persistence of the left anterior cardinal vein (which normally obliterates during embryogenesis) results in persistent left superior vena cava. LSVC drains via the coronary sinus to the right atrium in more than 90% of patients. Rarely, it may directly drain to the left atrium in association with other congenital heart defects (e.g. isomerism). Its prevalence is up to 0.5% in the general population, and higher in patients with congenital heart disease.

PFO
see patent foramen ovale.

phlebotomy
A palliative procedure involving withdrawal of whole blood (usually in up to 500 mL increments) which may be offered to patients with cyanotic CHD and secondary erythrocytosis who are experiencing hyperviscosity symptoms. Concomitant volume replacement is usually indicated.

pink tetralogy of Fallot
see tetralogy of Fallot.

polycythemia vera
A neoplastic transformation of all blood cell lines (erythrocyte, leukocyte, and platelet) associated with increased numbers of cells in the peripheral blood. Contrast with secondary erythrocytosis as seen in cyanotic heart disease. *see also* erythrocytosis.

polysplenia syndrome
see isomerism/left isomerism.

Potts shunt
A palliative operation for the purpose of increasing pulmonary blood flow, hence systemic oxygen saturation. The procedure involves creating a small communication between a pulmonary artery and the ipsilateral descending thoracic aorta. Often complicated by the development of pulmonary vascular obstructive disease if too large, or acquired stenosis or atresia of the pulmonary artery if distortion occurs. (Potts WJ, *et al.* Anastomosis of aorta to pulmonary artery: certain types of congenital heart disease. *Journal of the American Medical Association* 1946, **132**, 627–631.)

PPH
Primary pulmonary hypertension. see pulmonary hypertension.

probe-patent foramen ovale
see patent foramen ovale.

protein-losing enteropathy (PLE)
A complication seen following the Fontan operation in which protein is lost via the gut, resulting in ascites, peripheral edema, pleural and pericardial effusions. It is of unknown cause, though exacerbated by high systemic venous pressure. If serum protein and albumin are low, increased alpha-1 antitrypsin in the stool supports the diagnosis of PLE.

protrusio acetabulae
Abnormal displacement of the head of the femur within the acetabulum. A radiological finding useful in the diagnosis of Marfan syndrome.

pseudotruncus arteriosus
Pulmonary atresia with a VSD, biventricular aorta, and pulmonary blood flow provided by systemic to pulmonary collaterals. This anatomic arrangement had previously been called 'truncus arteriosus type IV' but is morphogenetically a different lesion from truncus arteriosus. In pseudotruncus, the single vessel arising from the ventricles is an aorta with an aortic valve, not a truncus with a truncal valve, and pulmonary blood flow derives from aorto-pulmonary collateral arteries, not from anomalously connected true pulmonary arteries.

pulmonary artery banding
Surgically created stenosis of the main pulmonary artery performed as a palliative procedure to protect the lungs against high blood flow and pressure when definitive correction of the underlying anomaly is not immediately advisable, e.g. in the setting of a non-restrictive VSD.

pulmonary artery sling
Anomalous origin of the left pulmonary artery from the right pulmonary artery, such that it loops around the trachea. It may be associated with complete cartilaginous rings in the distal trachea and tracheal stenosis. It may occur as an isolated entity or in association with other congenital heart defects.

pulmonary atresia
An imperforate pulmonary valve. When associated with a VSD (variant of tetralogy of Fallot), pulmonary blood flow arises from aorto-pulmonary collaterals, and systemic venous return exits the right heart via the VSD. When associated with intact interventricular septum, pulmonary artery blood supply is via a patent ductus arteriosus, and systemic venous return exits the right heart via an obligatory ASD.

pulmonary hypertension
Raised pulmonary arterial pressure. A common method to define the severity of pulmonary hypertension is the pulmonary/aortic systolic pressure ratio:

Severity	Ratio
mild	≥0.3, <0.6
moderate	≥0.6, <0.9
severe	≥0.9 (Eisenmenger syndrome)

Rashkind procedure

A balloon atrial septostomy performed as a palliative procedure in children with d-TGA. (Rashkind WJ, Miller WW. Creation of an atrial septal defect without thoracotomy: a palliative approach to complete transposition of the great arteries. *Journal of the American Medical Association* 1966, **196**, 991–992.)

Rastelli procedure (operation)

An operation for repair of complete transposition of the great arteries in association with a large VSD and pulmonic stenosis, wherein a communication is established between the left ventricle (LV) and the aorta via the VSD using a baffle within the right ventricle (RV). The RV is connected to the pulmonary artery using a valved conduit, and the LV-PA connection is obliterated. As a consequence, the left ventricle supports the systemic circulation. (Rastelli GC, *et al.* Anatomic correction of transposition of the great arteries with ventricular septal defect and subpulmonary stenosis. *Journal of Thoracic and Cardiovascular Surgery* 1969, **58**, 545–552.)

regional referral center (RRC)

A center for the care of adult patients with CHD, incorporating, at a minimum, cardiology staff with special skills, training, and experience in the management of such patients, and highly skilled echocardiographers.

restrictive right ventricular physiology

Physiologic behavior of the ventricles of some patients, e.g. after repair of tetralogy of Fallot. It may be defined by echocardiography as antegrade pulmonary artery flow in late diastole (a-wave) through all phases of respiration. The pulsed recordings are obtained with the sample volume at the midpoint between the pulmonary valve cusps or remnants and the pulmonary artery bifurcation. (Redington AN, *et al.* Antegrade diastolic pulmonary artery flow as a marker of right ventricular restriction after complete repair of pulmonary atresia with intact ventricular septum and critical pulmonary valve stenosis. *Cardiology in the Young* 1992, **2**, 382–386.)

restrictive VSD

see ventricular septal defect.

right aortic arch

see aortic arch anomalies.

right ventricular dysplasia

see Uhl anomaly.

Ross procedure
A method of aortic valve replacement involving autograft transplantation of the pulmonary valve, annulus and trunk into the aortic position, with reimplantation of the coronary ostia into the neo-aorta. The RVOT is reconstructed with a homograft conduit. (Ross DN. Replacement of aortic valve with a pulmonary autograft. *Lancet* 1967, **2**, 956–958.) (Ross D. Pulmonary valve autotransplantation [the Ross operation]. *Journal of Cardiac Surgery* 1988, **3**, 313–319.)

rubella syndrome
A wide spectrum of malformations caused by rubella infection early in pregnancy, including cataracts, retinopathy, deafness, congenital heart disease, bone lesions, mental retardation, etc. The spectrum of congenital heart lesions is wide and includes pulmonary artery stenosis, patent ductus arteriosus, tetralogy of Fallot, and ventricular septal defect.

Right ventricle (RV) infundibulum
A normal connecting segment between the body of the RV and the pulmonary artery. *syn.* RV conus. *see also* infundibulum.

RVOTO
Right ventricular outflow tract obstruction.

sail sound
An auscultatory finding in some patients with Ebstein anomaly. The S_1 includes mitral valve closure as its first component with a delayed tricuspid component. The abnormally large tricuspid anterior leaflet snapping like a sail catching the wind causes this delayed closure. The sail sound is not an ejection click, although it may simulate one.

scimitar syndrome
A constellation of anomalies including infradiaphragmatic total or partial anomalous pulmonary venous connection of the right lung to the inferior vena cava, often associated with hypoplasia of the right lung and right pulmonary artery (PA). The lower portion of the right lung tends to receive its arterial supply from the abdominal aorta. The name of the syndrome derives from the appearance on PA chest x-ray of the shadow formed by the anomalous pulmonary venous connection, which resembles a Turkish sword, or scimitar.

secondary erythrocytosis
see erythrocytosis. *see also* polycythemia vera.

Senning procedure (operation)
An operation for complete transposition of the great arteries in which venous return is directed to the contralateral ventricle by means of an atrial baffle fashioned in situ by using right atrial wall and interatrial septum. As a conse-

quence, the right ventricle supports the systemic circulation. A type of 'atrial switch' operation. *see also* Mustard procedure, atrial switch operation, double switch operation. (Senning A. Surgical correction of transposition of the great vessels. *Surgery* 1959, **45**, 966–980.)

Shone complex (syndrome)
An association of multiple levels of left ventricular inflow and outflow obstruction (subvalvar and valvar LVOTO, coarctation of the aorta and mitral stenosis [parachute mitral valve and supramitral ring]). (Shone JD, *et al.* The developmental complex of 'parachute mitral valve', supravalvular ring of left atrium, subaortic stenosis and coarctation of aorta. *American Journal of Cardiology* 1963, **11**, 714–725.)

Shprintzen syndrome
see velo-cardio-facial syndrome. *see* CATCH 22.

shunt
Movement of blood through a congenitally abnormal or surgically created connection and communication between two circuits, at the level of the atria, ventricles, or great vessels. 'Shunt' is a physiologic term, in contrast to 'connection' which is an anatomic term.

single (as in atrium, ventricle, etc.)
Implies absence of the corresponding contralateral structure. Contrasts with 'common', which implies bilateral structures with absent septation. *see also* common.

sinus venosus
An embryologic structure, the anatomic precursor of the inferior vena cava, superior vena cava and coronary sinus and part of the definitive right atrium, which is located external to the primitive right atrium in the early embryologic period (3 to 4 weeks' gestation). The sinus portion of the right atrium receives the inferior vena cava, superior vena cava and coronary sinus. The right and left valves of the sinus venosus separate the sinus venosus from the primitive right atrium, the embryologic precursor of the trabeculated or muscular portion of the right atrium, and includes the right atrial appendage, which in turn communicates with the tricuspid valve. The left valve of the sinus venosus joins the interatrial septum, retrogresses and is absorbed. The right valve of the sinus venosus enlarges and functions to deflect the oxygenated fetal blood coming from the placenta and via the inferior vena cava across the foramen ovale. *see also* cor triatriatum dexter, sinus venosus defect.

sinus venosus defect
A communication located postero-superior (or rarely postero-inferior) to the oval fossa, commonly associated with partial anomalous pulmonary venous

connection (most often right pulmonary veins, especially the right upper pulmonary vein in association with a postero-superior defect), which is functionally identical to an atrial septal defect, but properly named a sinus venosus defect because it occurs due to abnormal development of the sinus venosus in relation to the pulmonary veins and is not a defect in the interatrial septum. *see also* atrial septal defect

situs
syn. sidedness. The position of the morphologic right atrium determines the sidedness and is independent of the direction of the cardiac apex, or the positions of the ventricles or the great arteries.
• situs ambiguous. Indeterminate sidedness (in the setting of atrial isomerism).
• situs inversus. Mirror-image sidedness, i.e. opposite of normal. Left-sided morphologic right atrium.
• situs inversus totalis. Total mirror-image sidedness. The position of all lateralized organs is inverted.
• situs solitus. Normal sidedness. Right-sided morphologic right atrium.

stent
Intravascular (intraluminal) prosthesis to scaffold a vessel following transluminal balloon dilatation, for the purpose of maintaining patency.

Sterling Edwards procedure
A palliative operation for transposition of the great arteries in which the atrial septum was resected, repositioned, and sutured to the left of the right pulmonary veins to produce drainage into the right atrium. The procedure produced left-to-right shunt of oxygenated blood directly into the systemic atrium and ventricle and offloaded the pulmonary circulation in patients with complete transposition of the great arteries and high pulmonary flow. (Edwards WS, Bargeron LM, *et al.* Reposition of right pulmonary veins in transposition of the great vessels. *Journal of the American Medical Association* 1964, **188**, 522–523. Edwards WS, Bargeron LM. More effective palliation of the transposition of the great vessels. *Journal of Thoracic and Cardiovascular Surgery* 1965, **19**, 790–795.)

straddling AV valve
see atrioventricular valve.

subpulmonary ventricle
The ventricle that relates most directly to the pulmonary artery.

supero-inferior heart
A term applied to a heart the ventricles of which are in a markedly supero-inferior relationship due to abnormal displacement of the ventricular mass along the horizontal plane of its long axis. Often coexists with criss-cross atrioven-

tricular relationships. *see also* criss-cross heart. *syn.* over-and-under ventricles; upstairs-downstairs heart.

supracristal
Located above the crista supraventricularis in the right ventricular outflow tract, hence contiguous with the origin of the great arteries. see crista supraventricularis.

supraregional referral center (SRRC)
A 'full service' center for providing optimal care of adult patients with CHD comprising specialized resources, the availability of cardiology specialists with specific training and experience in ACHD, the availability of other cardiology sub-specialists and other medical and paramedical personnel with special training/experience in the problems of congenital heart disease, and offering opportunities for training, research and education in the field. *syn.* national referral center.

supravalvar mitral ring
An anomaly found in the left atrium that produces congenital mitral stenosis. *see also* cor triatriatum. *see also* Shone complex.

switch-conversion of transposition
An operation performed in patients with congenitally corrected transposition of the great arteries, or in patients who had previously had a Mustard or Senning procedure for complete transposition of the great arteries, to allow the left ventricle to assume the function of the systemic ventricle. The first stage may involve pulmonary artery banding to induce pulmonary left ventricular hypertrophy. The second stage involves an arterial switch operation in both groups and a Mustard or Senning operation in patients with congenitally corrected transposition, or removal of the Mustard/Senning atrial baffles and reconstruction of an atrial septum in patients with complete TGA. *see also* double switch operation.

systemic AV valve
The atrioventricular valve guarding the inlet to the systemic ventricle.

TAPVC
Total anomalous pulmonary venous connection. *see* anomalous pulmonary venous connection.

TAPVD
Total anomalous pulmonary venous drainage. A term sometimes used to refer to the entity properly called total anomalous pulmonary venous connection. *see* anomalous pulmonary venous connection.

Taussig-Bing anomaly
A form of double outlet right ventricle in which the great arteries arise side-by-side with the aorta to the right of the pulmonary artery and the ventricular septal defect in a subpulmonary position. Since the left ventricle empties across the VSD preferentially into the pulmonary artery, the physiology simulates complete transposition of the great arteries with a VSD.

tetralogy of Fallot
A congenital anomaly, the primary pathophysiologic components of which are obstruction to right ventricular outflow at the infundibular level and a large nonrestrictive VSD. The other two components of the 'tetralogy' are an overriding aorta and concentric right ventricular hypertrophy. Valvar RVOTO (pulmonic stenosis) and distal pulmonary artery stenosis are often present. The essential morphogenetic anomaly is malalignment of the infundibular (outlet) septum such that it fails to unite with the trabecular septum (hence the VSD) due to anterior deviation (hence the RVOTO). Lillehei first described the repair in 1955. (Lillehei CW, *et al*. Direct vision intracardiac surgical correction of the tetralogy of Fallot, pentalogy of Fallot, and pulmonary atresia defects; reports of first ten cases. *Annals of Surgery* 1955, **142**, 418–445.)
• pentalogy of Fallot. Tetralogy of Fallot with an associated ASD or PFO.
• pink tetralogy of Fallot. Tetralogy of Fallot presenting with increased pulmonary blood flow and minimal cyanosis because of a lesser degree of RVOTO. *syn*. acyanotic Fallot.

Thebesian valve
A remnant of the right valve of the sinus venosus guarding the opening of the coronary sinus.

total anomalous pulmonary venous connection (drainage, return)
see anomalous pulmonary venous connection/total anomalous pulmonary venous connection.

trabecular VSD
see ventricular septal defect

transannular
Crossing the annulus. In connection with the RVOT in tetralogy of Fallot, the term refers to the pulmonary valve annulus, which often must be enlarged by a transannular patch, with consequent obligatory pulmonary insufficiency. Transannular patching was first described in 1959. (Kirklin JW, *et al*. Surgical treatment for tetralogy of Fallot by open intracardiac repair. *Journal of Thoracic Surgery* 1959, **37**, 22–51.)

transposition of the great arteries (TGA)

see discordant ventriculo-arterial connections and see below

- simple TGA. Discordant connection of the great arteries and ventricles such that the pulmonary trunk arises from the left ventricle and the aorta arises from the right ventricle, without any associated abnormality.
- complex transposition of the great arteries. Discordant connection of the great arteries and ventricles such that the pulmonary trunk arises from the left ventricle and the aorta arises from the right ventricle, with associated abnormalities, most commonly a ventricular septal defect.

tricuspid atresia

A congenital anomaly in which there is no physiologic or gross morphologic connection between the right atrium and right ventricle, and there is an inter-atrial connection allowing mixing of systemic and pulmonary venous return at the atrial level. There is a variable degree of hypoplasia of the right ventricle. The left ventricle and mitral valve are normal.

truncus arteriosus

A single artery (truncus) arises from the base of the heart because of failure of proximal division into the aorta and the pulmonary artery. Thus, both pulmonary and systemic arteries as well as the coronary arteries arise from the common trunk. Truncus arteriosus is divided into two types depending on whether there is a VSD or an intact ventricular septum. *syn.* common arterial trunk.

Turner syndrome

A clinical syndrome due to the 45 XO karyotype in about 50% of cases, with 45XO/45XX mosaicism and other X chromosome abnormalities comprising the remainder. There is a characteristic but variable phenotype, and association with congenital cardiac anomalies, especially post-ductal coarctation of the aorta and other left-sided obstructive lesions, as well as partial anomalous pulmonary venous drainage without ASD. The female phenotype varies with the age of presentation, and is somewhat similar to that of Noonan syndrome.

Uhl anomaly

Congenital malformation consisting of nearly total absence of the right ventricular myocardium, presenting with marked enlargement of both the right ventricle and right atrium and subsequent tricuspid regurgitation. Arrhythmogenic right ventricular cardiomyopathy may be one end of a spectrum and Uhl anomaly the other.

unbalanced AV canal

see ventricular imbalance.

unifocalization
A surgical technique that creates a common trunk for multiple direct aorto-pulmonary collateral arteries, as part of the surgical management of complex pulmonary atresia.

univentricular connection
Both atria are connected to only one ventricle. The connection is univentricular, but the heart is usually biventricular.

unroofed coronary sinus
An anomaly in which there is a deficiency in the normal separation of the coronary sinus from the left atrium as the coronary sinus passes behind the left atrium (LA) in the AV groove, such that the coronary sinus drains into the LA. A form of absence of the coronary sinus.

upstairs-downstairs heart
see supero-inferior heart.

VACTERL association
Describes a spectrum of defects including vertebral abnormalities, anal atresia, tracheo-esophageal fistula, radial dysplasia, renal abnormalities and congenital heart defects (atrial and ventricular septal defect, tetralogy of Fallot, truncus arteriosus, aortic coarctation, patent ductus arteriosus, etc.).

vascular ring
A wide spectrum of aortic arch anomalies including double aortic arch and other vascular structures that surround the trachea and the esophagus resulting in their compression. The vascular structures may or may not be patent. Vascular rings may be isolated (in 1% to 2% of CHD) or associated with other CHD malformations, such as tetralogy of Fallot. *see* aortic arch anomalies.

velo-cardio-facial syndrome
Syndrome of cleft palate, abnormal facies (square nasal root, long nose with narrow alar base, long face with malar hypoplasia, long philtrum, thickened helix, low set ears), velopharyngeal incompetence and congenital cardiac defects (cono-truncal anomalies, isolated VSD, tetralogy of Fallot). Due to micro-deletion at chromosome 22q11. *syn.* Shprintzen syndrome. *see also* CATCH 22.

venous (or pulmonary) AV valve
The AV valve guarding the inlet to the venous, or pulmonary, ventricle.

ventricle repair
• 1-ventricle repair. *see* Fontan operation
• 1.5-ventricle repair (one and one-half ventricle repair). A term used to describe operations for cyanotic congenital heart disease performed when the pulmonary ventricle is insufficiently developed to accept the entire systemic

venous return. A bidirectional cavopulmonary connection is constructed to divert superior vena cava flow directly to the lungs, while inferior vena cava flow is directed to the lungs via the functioning but small pulmonary ventricle.

• 2-ventricle repair. A term used to describe operations for cyanotic congenital heart disease with common ventricle wherein functioning systemic and pulmonary ventricles are created by means of surgical septation of the common ventricle.

ventricular imbalance

In the setting of atrioventricular septal defect, ventricular imbalance refers to relative hypoplasia of one or the other of the ventricles in association with small size of the ipsilateral component of the atrioventricular annulus.

ventricular septal defect (VSD)

A defect in the ventricular septum, such that there is direct communication between the two ventricles.

• doubly-committed VSD. A defect in the outlet septum such that there is fibrous continuity between the aortic and pulmonary valves, with the VSD situated directly beneath both semilunar valves.

• inlet VSD. A defect in the lightly trabeculated inlet portion of the muscular interventricular septum, typically seen as part of an atrioventricular septal defect.

• muscular VSD. A defect entirely surrounded by muscular interventricular septum.

• nonrestrictive VSD. A ventricular septal defect of such a size that there is no significant pressure gradient between the ventricles. Hence, the pulmonary artery is exposed to systemic pressure unless there is RVOTO.

• outlet VSD. A defect in the non-trabeculated outlet portion of the muscular interventricular septum, hence above the crista supraventricularis. *syn.* supracristal VSD. Sometimes also described as subpulmonary, subarterial, or doubly committed subarterial VSD.

• perimembranous VSD. A VSD located in the membranous portion of the interventricular septum with variable extension into the contiguous portions of the inlet, trabecular, or outlet portions of the muscular septum, but not involving the atrioventricular septum. *syn.* membranous VSD; infracristal VSD.

• restrictive VSD. A ventricular septal defect of small enough size that there is a pressure gradient between the ventricles, such that the pulmonary ventricle (hence pulmonary vasculature) is protected from the systemic pressure of the contralateral ventricle.

• trabecular VSD. A defect in the heavily trabeculated central or trabecular portion of the muscular interventricular septum. May be multiple.

ventriculo-arterial concordance

see concordant ventriculo-arterial connections.

ventriculo-arterial discordance
see discordant ventriculo-arterial connections.

Waterston shunt
A palliative operation for the purpose of increasing pulmonary blood flow, hence systemic oxygen saturation, which involves creating a small communication between the main pulmonary artery and the ascending aorta. Often complicated by the development of pulmonary vascular obstructive disease if too large. Not uncommonly caused distortion of the pulmonary artery. (Waterston DJ. Treatment of Fallot's tetralogy in children under one year of age. *Rozhl Chir* 1962, **41**, 181–183.)

Williams syndrome
An autosomal dominant syndrome, often arising de novo, associated with an abnormality of elastin, infantile hypercalcemia, mild cognitive impairment and the so-called 'cocktail personality', and congenital heart disease, especially supravalvar aortic stenosis and multiple peripheral pulmonary stenoses. (Williams JC, *et al*. Supravalvular aortic stenosis. *Circulation* 1961, **24**, 1311–1318.) (Beuren A, *et al*. Supravalvular aortic stenosis in association with mental retardation and certain facial features. *Circulation* 1962, **26**, 1235–1240.)

Wolff-Parkinson-White (WPW) syndrome
Accessory lateral atrioventricular conduction pathway causing characteristic EKG changes and atrial (and sometimes ventricular) arrhythmias. WPW syndrome may be isolated or associated with congenital heart defects. It is found in up to 25% of patients with Ebstein anomaly. Typically, they have more than one accessory pathway.

Wood unit
A non-standard unit for expressing pulmonary vascular resistance (mmHg/L), named after Paul Wood, the famous British cardiologist. One Wood unit is equivalent to 80 dyn.cm.sec^{-5}.

xenograft
Tissue or organ used for transplant, derived from another species. *syn*. Heterograft.

Z-score, Z-value
A way of expressing a physiologic variable in a form corrected for age and body size. Important in pediatrics. This is the number of standard deviations a measurement departs from mean normal. (Rimoldi HJA, *et al*. A note on the concept of normality and abnormality in quantitation of pathologic findings in congenital heart disease. *Pediatric Clinics of North America* 1963, **10**, 589–591.) (Daubeney PEF, *et al*. Relationship of the dimension of cardiac structures to body size: an echocardiographic study in normal infants and children. *Cardiology in the Young* 1999, **9**, 402–410.)

Appendix: Shunt Calculations

Craig Broberg, MD, Senior Fellow in
Adult Congenital Heart Disease, Royal Brompton Hospital,
London, UK

Background

Despite the emergence of echo Doppler and MRI techniques for determining flow, catheterization-based studies remain the accepted clinical standard to quantify flow, particularly in patients with intracardiac shunts. The severity and significance of the shunt, and thus decisions about intervention, are often made based upon these calculations.

Although several potential tools are available in the catheterization laboratory, such as indicator dilution, by far the most commonly accepted is oximetry data applied to the Fick principle. However, the method makes multiple assumptions about oxygen content, physiologic stability, and mixing of shunted blood, which must be understood (Hillis *et al.*, 1985). This brief outline reviews the calculations involved and points out some of the potential sources for error using this method.

An online calculator with these same functions is now available (http://www.rbh.nthames.nhs.uk/cardiology/flowcalculations.asp).

Data required

1 Hemoglobin (Hgb in g/dl).
2 Oxygen consumption (VO_2 in ml/min): Best if measured by an oxygen sensor at the time of catheterization. Often assumed based on samples from the population available in the literature (LaFarge & Miettinen, 1970), for example:
    (a) Women: $VO_2 = BSA \times [138.1 - 17.04 \times \ln(age) + 0.378 \times HR]$
    (b) Men: $VO_2 = BSA \times [138.1 - 11.49 \times \ln(age) + 0.378 \times HR]$
3 Percentage oxygen saturation from the following:
    (a) Mixed venous (MV_{sat}): multiple ways of determining MV_{sat} based on SVC_{sat} and IVC_{sat} exist. One standard approach is to use the SVC value alone as the mixed venous, since it approximates the average between IVC (renal blood is less desaturated) and coronary sinus (coronary blood is more desaturated). Alternatively, one calculates an average based on any of the following formulae (Flamm *et al.*, 1970; French *et al.*, 1983; Pirwitz *et al.*, 1997):
      (i) $MV_{sat} = [(SVC_{sat} \times 3) + IVC_{sat}]/4$
      (ii) $MV_{sat} = [(SVC_{sat}) + (IVC_{sat} \times 2)]/3$
      (iii) $MV_{sat} = [(SVC_{sat} \times 2) + (IVC_{sat} \times 3)]/5$

(b) Pulmonary artery (PA_{sat}): usually obtained from the main pulmonary artery. Optimally should be sampled from right and left pulmonary arteries selectively and averaged, particularly if a patent ductus arteriosus is present.

(c) Pulmonary venous (PV_{sat}): can be obtained often through an atrial septal defect or patent foramen ovale. Different pulmonary veins may have different values, due to degree of ventilatory mismatch (Iga *et al.*, 1999). Thus, a mixed value, such as left atrial saturation, may be the purest site to sample if there is no shunting at the atrial level.

(d) Aortic saturation (Ao_{sat}): can be measured directly from anywhere in the aorta, often sampled from the femoral artery. Percutaneous oxygen saturation can substitute with reasonable accuracy, though not if a patent ductus arteriosus is present.

Formulae

Flow calculations are based on the Fick principle as follows:

$$\text{Flow} = \frac{\text{oxygen consumption (VO}_2)}{(\text{proximal oxygen content}) - (\text{distal oxygen content})}$$

Oxygen content is O_2 carrying capacity multiplied by O_2 saturation.

1 Calculate O_2 carrying capacity as follows:

$$O_{2capacity} = Hgb \times 1.36 \times 10$$

2 Blood flow (Q) in L/min:
  (a) $Q_{pulmonic} = VO_2/[O_{2capacity} \times (PV_{sat} - PA_{sat})/100]$
  (b) $Q_{systemic} = VO_2/[O_{2capacity} \times (Ao_{sat} - MV_{sat})/100]$
  (c) Effective flow is the amount of non-shunted flow carried from systemic to pulmonic capillary beds:

$$Q_{effective} = VO_2/[O_{2capacity} \times (PV_{sat} - MV_{sat})/100]$$

3 Shunt volumes in L/min:
  (a) Right-to-left shunt = $Q_{systemic} - Q_{effective}$
  (b) Left-to-right shunt = $Q_{pulmonic} - Q_{effective}$
4 Flow/shunt fractions:
  (a) $Q_{pulmonic}/Q_{systemic}$ (Qp/Qs)

$$= \frac{Ao_{sat} - MV_{sat}}{PV_{sat} - PA_{sat}}$$

(b) Pulmonic shunt fraction (the fraction of pulmonic flow due to left to right shunting)

$$= \frac{PA_{sat} - MV_{sat}}{PV_{sat} - MV_{sat}}$$

(c) Systemic shunt fraction (the fraction of systemic flow due to right to left shunting)

$$= \frac{PV_{sat} - Ao_{sat}}{PV_{sat} - MV_{sat}}$$

Potential sources of error

1 *Oximetry measurement*: small errors in saturation measurement can produce large errors in Qp/Qs (Cigarroa *et al.*, 1989; Shepherd *et al.*, 1997). Saturations can either be measured using spectrophotometry or by obtaining PO_2 by blood gas analysis and calculating SaO_2 using the oxygen-hemoglobin dissociation curve. Spectrophotometry can be erroneous in patients with carboxyhemoglobin or hyperbilirubinemia. Blood gas analysis data can be wrong in conditions where there might be a significant shift in the dissociation curve, such as anemia and other metabolic derangements. Patients with chronic cyanotic heart disease often have a shift in this dissociation curve. Incomplete wasting before obtaining samples also results in error.

2 *Supplemental oxygen*: usually, the amount of dissolved oxygen in the blood is negligible in the above calculations, but this will not be the case if the patient is on high amounts of supplemental oxygen. In fact, placing the patient on oxygen is sometimes done to improve the calculations. If so, samples should be measured using blood gas analyzer, and the oxygen content for each condition should be recalculated as follows (where PO_2 is given in mmHg):

$$O_2 \text{ content} = (O_{2capacity} \times SaO_2) + (PO_2 \times 0.003)$$

3 *High flow states*: in high flow states, mixed venous oxygen saturation is higher, and thus sensitivity of shunt detection is lower.

4 Many reported historical values and tables for VO_2 are based on normal, sedated individuals and thus are not representative of patients. Every patient will have variation in oxygen consumption on a minute-to-minute basis. Thus, data should be obtained as quickly as possible, preferably on pullback, and should be obtained in quiet, resting, controlled conditions.

References

Cigarroa RG, Lange RA & Hillis LD (1989) Oximetric quantitation of intracardiac left-to-right shunting: limitations of the Qp/Qs ratio. *American Journal of Cardiology*, **64**, 246–247.

Flamm MD, Cohn KE & Hancock EW (1970) Ventricular function in atrial septal defect. *American Journal of Medicine*, **48**, 286–294.

French WJ, Chang P, Forsythe S & Criley JM (1983) Estimation of mixed venous oxygen saturation. *Catheter Cardiovascular Diagnosis*, **9**, 25–31.

Hillis LD, Winniford MD, Jackson JA & Firth BG (1985) Measurements of left-to-right intracardiac shunting in adults: oximetric versus indicator dilution techniques. *Catheter Cardiovascular Diagnosis*, **11**, 467–472.

Iga K, Izumi C, Matsumura M, *et al.* (1999) Partial pressure of oxygen is lower in the left upper pulmonary vein than in the right in adults with atrial septal defect: difference in $P(O_2)$ between the right and left pulmonary veins. *Chest*, **115**, 679–683.

LaFarge CG & Miettinen OS (1970) The estimation of oxygen consumption. *Cardiovascular Research*, **4**, 23–30.

Pirwitz MJ, Willard JE, Landau C, Hillis LD & Lange RA (1997) A critical reappraisal of the oximetric assessment of intracardiac left-to-right shunting in adults. *American Heart Journal*, **133**, 413–417.

Shepherd AP, Steinke JM & McMahan CA (1997) Effect of oximetry error on the diagnostic value of the Qp/Qs ratio. *International Journal of Cardiology*, **61**, 247–259.

Index

Page numbers in *italics* refer to figures and those in **bold** to tables; but note that figures and tables are only indicated when they are separated from their text references.